Praise for *IN HER OWN WORDS*:

"*In Her Own Words* is personal, emotional and insightful. Fran Lewis shares intimate details of a family's story and offers valuable words of advice. This is a must read for anyone whose life has been touched by Alzheimer's."

— Michael Tabman, Retired FBI Agent, Author of *Midnight Sin*, *Bad Intent* and *Walking the Corporate Beat*

"*In Her Own Words* is at once harrowing, inspiring and engrossing. An emotional journey that also provides practical and crucial information for care-givers."

— Dennis Palumbo, MFT, licensed psychotherapist and author

In Her Own Words is a must read for everyone. It presents in a compelling and compassionate way, the evolution of Alzheimer's from the standpoint of Fran's mother. At the same time, it focuses with empathy and insight on the caregiver. This book contains objective medical information on symptoms and behavior. I would strongly recommend *In Her Own Words* by Fran Lewis because unfortunately, this disease could strike anyone.

— Best Selling and award winning author of *The Argentine Triangle* and *The Russian Endgame,* Allan Topol

Praise for *IN HER OWN WORDS*:

"Thank you so much for sharing the story with me. Not only was it a poignant story, but it was so helpful!

"I was especially moved by the portion from your mom's point of view on what her day is like (Life as I see it now). Wow, that was excellent writing. But beyond being informative, the information and advice about being a health care provider is so very valuable.

"I loved reading the anecdotes and the poems. Also, it was fascinating learning about her mom and step mom and of course her relationship with you. That history was so impactful because I felt I had really known your mom. So when I was reading about this illness, it was someone I knew already, and admired.

"The story is a wonderful tribute. Her life was important to the people who knew and loved her, but thanks to your efforts, her life will be important to many others. Is this book the same as on your Amazon page titled *Memories Are Precious*? If so, I would be happy and honored to review it. Thanks again for sharing and especially for writing the story."

— Ben Lieberman, author of *The Carnage Account* and *Odd Jobs*

"Fran Lewis has written a wonderful book that will enlighten readers as to what really happens to the person suffering from Alzheimer disease and their family. This horrible battle they fight must not go unnoticed. Families face challenges they never imagined in their wildest dreams and when they read this book they will know they are not alone. Fran maps out exactly what happened to her family hoping that others may be spared some of the traumatic occurrences. *In Her Own Words* is quite a story and very special. Fran, your mother was very lucky to have you by her side in both good and difficult times. "

— Marsha Casper Cook, Michigan Avenue Media Inc.

Praise for *IN HER OWN WORDS*:

"In Her Own Words by Fran Lewis is the book about Alzheimer's disease we've all been waiting for without knowing it.

As the title indicates, it is the patient herself, Ruth Swerdloff, who dominates the narrative. Shown as a woman with a regular family history, a 'normal' life and unrelated health problems we get to see what is important in her life, what she cares for and what she is like.

Then we accompany her on her gruesome journey from early signs of the disease, to diagnosis, to deterioration and care.

This is a story that spares nothing: not the pain, no detail of the struggle with dignity and control. Swerdloff and Lewis tell it like it is. Without cover-ups and pretence we get to witness what it is really like to live with the disease and care for someone who suffers from it.

There is plenty of added information from the author about all the little and big things everyone needs to know and what caring for someone who is affected by it truly involves. From the formal to the mundane, from official to personal – Lewis has lived through it and seems to have thought of everything there is to know and to ask.

A book both heart-breaking and inspiring because Lewis provides the reader with so many thoughtful and useful tips and ideas as how to come to terms with the situation and best handle it. And the way the family cared for Ruth is amazing and shows that this can be done.

I strongly recommend you read this. And important, informative and inspiring story that will pull on your heartstrings but will leave you with knowledgeable and for-armed.

Highly recommended.

— Christoph Fischer, author of *Conditions*

THE VANISHING MIND OF RUTH SWERDLOFF

IN HER OWN WORDS

An Alzheimer's Sufferer's Journal

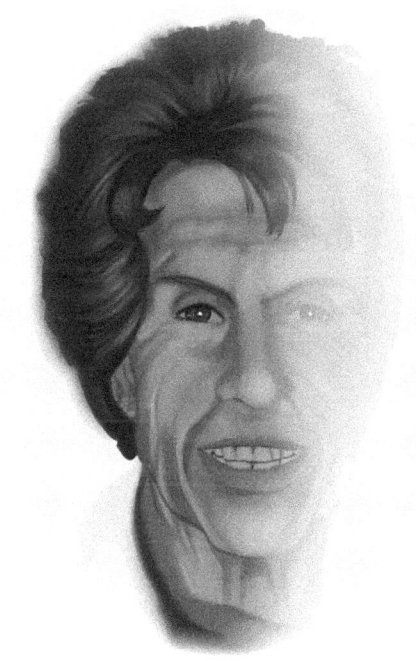

WRITTEN BY

FRAN LEWIS

PUBLISHED BY FIDELI PUBLISHING INC.

ISBN: 978-1-60414-848-0

Published by:
Fideli Publishing, Inc.
119 W. Morgan St.
Martinsville, IN 46151

www.FideliPublishing.com

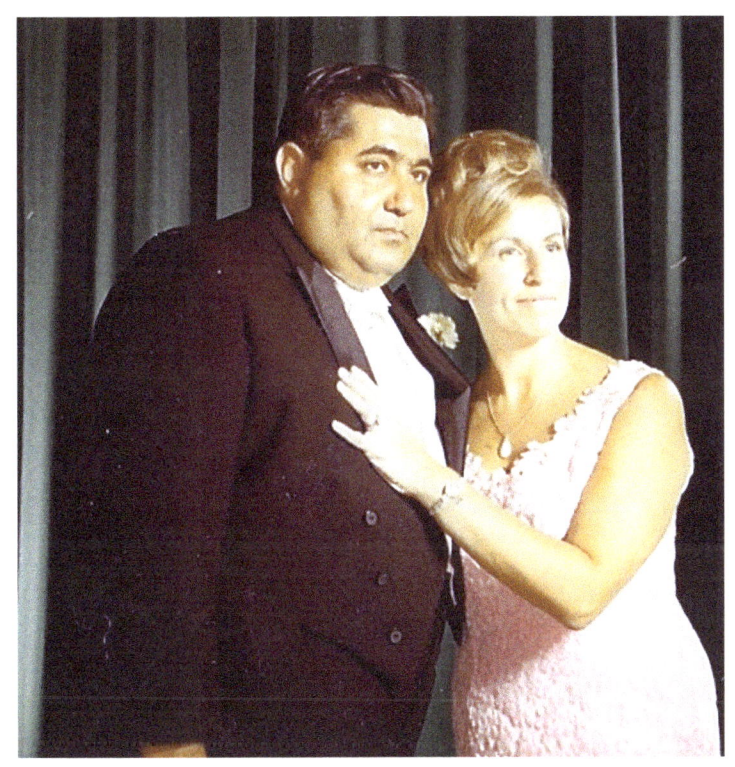

Dedicated to my mom, Ruth Swerdloff,
a truly remarkable woman

Contents

PART ONE
An Alzheimer's Sufferer's Journal

CHAPTER ONE
How It All Began

CHAPTER TWO
Things Aren't Quite Right

CHAPTER THREE
The Diagnosis

CHAPTER FOUR
The Uninvited Guest

CHAPTER FIVE
Becoming the Caregiver

CHAPTER SIX
The Harsh Truth Sets In

CHAPTER SEVEN
Ruth's Final Chapter

PART FOUR
Family Memories

Acknowledgments

I want to thank all of the members of my family who wrote dedications to family members or friends, and helped contribute to making this book and project successful.

I also want to thank all of the authors and my close friends for their dedications and memories, too. I want to personally thank the following authors for their help: Carla Neggers, Dennis Palumbo, Larry Thompson, Susan Ross, Michael Tabman, Allan Topol, Marsha Cook and Christoph Fischer.

Thank you to Dr. Joel Cohen for the love and support you gave my mom and my family when you realized how seriously ill my mom was. Thank you for always answering our cries for help and always being there when we needed you. You are truly a rare and special doctor, and a caring and understanding person.

Finally, I want to thank my family for their support, especially my sister Marcia, who thought right from the start this was a great way to let people know about our mom and about the urgent need to find a cure for Alzheimer's disease.

From the Author

Within the pages of this book you will hear my mom's own words, which I have not edited. You might find some expressions, typos or syntax errors in her stories. I purposely left them so that everyone will understand what she went through and how her language patterns changed during the course of her journey with this dreaded illness.

My mom was brave, courageous and strong-willed and never gave up on life or herself. I added information for caregivers, families, aides, friends, nursing agencies, RNs, CNRs, medical staff and anyone that might be caring for someone with this illness. You will hear her words, read stories that she dictated to me to put into her journal, my sister's thoughts and the thoughts of family members that want you to know her before was she was diagnosed.

She always knew who she was and where she lived. She remembered her children, though not always by name but by facial recognition. Her name was Ruth and this is her story!

Introduction

The purpose of this book is to make people aware of the need for a cure for Alzheimer's disease. This deadly disease has taken too many lives in the 103 years since Dr. Alois Alzheimer discovered it in 1906.

Presently, Alzheimer's is not curable. There are no real medications to slow down what happens to those who are afflicted. My mom took two different types of medication, and neither worked to slow down the progression of the disease.

I have learned in the past twelve years that there are many important things everyone should know about getting care for their loved one or themselves before the disease finally takes over and the individual cannot make the decisions themselves.

The book tells my mom's story in her words from the day she found out she had Alzheimer's disease. I have also included tips for caregivers, like myself, as well as a list of what medical services are available and how to get them and information on the stages of the disease, and what legal documents need to be filed and prepared. There are also dedications from family members, short anecdotes about times they spent with her, and more.

This information targets all segments of the population, in the hope that it will be used as an educational tool. I think young children and teens, as well as all adults need to have a full understanding of Alzheimer's disease and how it affects everyone in the patient's family. It can destroy relationships, and put both mental and physical stress on the person who has taken on the role of caregiver. The book includes information to help the caregiver deal with this stress and take care of him or herself.

Foreword

Alzheimer's disease took my mom's mind slowly, and on March 7, 2011 it took her life. She fought long and hard to remain in this world, never once giving up on herself. She realized, in her own way, that what happened to her was not her fault and that disease would impact everyone's lives.

Alzheimer's disease is a deadly illness with no cure. Those with the responsibility of caregiver need to realize what they are undertaking, and also be aware that they might be in this alone. Caregivers might find that someone will give them a temporary respite, but in my experience that didn't occur very often. The caregiver's lives will be greatly curtailed and their alone time limited, but the fact that they kept someone alive with their care is all that really matters.

In my mother's case, the cost of home health aides put me in great debt. Never considering what it would take financially to pay for the aides' time before getting full Medicaid, I just went ahead and agreed to make sure my mom received the best 24-hour care from four of the best home care aides in the world. Knowing what I know now, would I do it again? In a heartbeat. She is the reason I have a great work ethic, enjoy reading and reviewing books, love doing radio, and remember the importance of family.

This is really *our* true story into this wasteland of horror. While I find it painful to retell, it needs to be told so that everyone understands how serious the disease is, and how important it is to help the loved one with this diagnosis. Take the journey with my mother, my family and me as she gets the diagnosis that will forever change all our lives and reduce her from a productive, vibrant person to nothing.

An Alzheimer's Sufferer's Journal

How It All Began

Meet Ruth Swerdloff — 2002

The following was created from the personal journals my mother, Ruth, kept from the moment she realized something was wrong. The text from her journals will be indented and presented in a different typeface so that you will recognize it. These entries are exact duplicates of her journal. Any grammar errors, discrepancies and other oddities are included to illustrate her mental decline.

Ruth wanted everyone to get to know her as a person, so she started with a brief description of her life after the diagnosis.

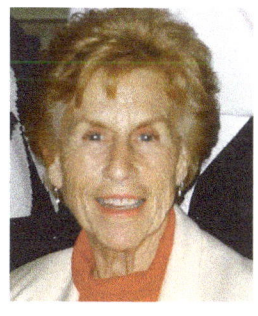

> My name is Ruth Swerdloff, and I was born on November 22, 1927 to Max and Fanny Goldberg. Fanny, my mom, was a special person. She spoke five languages and had five children that she loved dearly. Unfortunately, I never really got to know her. She died when I was two after giving birth to a sixth child. She died of pneumonia.

> Having five children and believing that children needed a mother, my dad, Max Jacob Goldberg, decided to find a mother for his five children, but in a very special and old-

fashioned way. Fanny had sisters named Rosie, Tillie, Katie, and Shondina. Each was unique and special in her own way. Shondina was not a very friendly person, and Tillie was a tad spoiled and needed to be taken care of. Rosie was great, but she was married to my Uncle Dave at the time. So, my father decided to choose from the other three sisters which one Fanny, my mom, would want to bring up her five children.

Three months after her death my father married Katie. Katie was the only mother that I ever knew, and she was the most amazing, unselfish, smart, and perfect choice to be the mother of five not-so-easy-to-handle kids. There was Tova, my sister, who was ten years older than me. Then there was Irving, Harry, and Kenny. They gave her a really hard time at first because they were old enough to know their real mother, and thought that my dad should have waited before taking a new wife. But, my father was the smartest man in the world and he made the best and wisest choice, not only in picking a new wife but in business too.

I never knew that Katie was not my real mother until much later. I lived on Southern Boulevard and Tremont Avenue. I went to P.S. 44 and Roosevelt High School. I adored my mom and I could not understand what the other kids in my family had a problem with until later on when I found out the truth.

Growing up I was always closest to my brother Kenny. As the youngest in the family, I can say that I was a tad spoiled and could do no wrong. I loved to dance and wanted to be a Rockette when I grew up. I also loved twirling a baton, and I did become a drum majorette in high school.

I never knew or thought that what would happen to me in later life would ever come to pass. I never heard of Alzheimer's disease or even dementia. No one in my family ever had a memory problem or anything close to it. As a matter of fact my mother and father never forgot anything, and neither did my brothers or sister.

Tova was a teacher, and graduated college when she was sixteen years old. You might say she was a genius and could do anything, and could remember things after reading them only once. Kenny went into the army and fought in the Second World War. Irving and Harry were very smart, but due to the depression and hard times it was hard to get jobs, and my dad had to figure out a way to help his children when they graduated school to make a living.

When my father came to America he landed on Ellis Island. He brought his family to live in the Bronx and sold apples on a street corner for a living. Being extremely enterprising, he managed to make enough money to buy a Laundromat and then a cleaning store on 180th Street and Mohegan Avenue. He named the store Arista Cleaners. Arista in school meant the highest, and was an organization that the smartest kids, who had over ninety averages, were inducted in. Arista Cleaners was the best cleaning store with the highest standards in cleaning and the best customer service. All of my brothers worked there, and my sister taught in P.S. 67 in the Bronx.

Katie, our mom, was the most amazing woman. She took care of us as if we were her very own children. I know that she even adopted all five of us, but I was too young at the time to know that. When I found out I was devastated. I was walking home with my cousin from the movies and I realized that I was going to be late. I told her that my mother would be upset, and she said "Why do you care? She is not your real mother." She proceeded to explain.

I went into our small apartment and into my room, and cried for hours and hours. I never told anyone that I knew the truth, and I made my cousin swear that she would never tell anyone that she told me. Until the day she died, my mother, Katie, never knew that I found out she was not my real mother. I would never hurt her.

She was so smart and could do anything. She was in a concentration camp in Poland during the First World War and was tortured. They were experimenting with x-rays, and as a result she became sterile and could not have any children. She had other problems because of this. She was practically blind in both eyes due to cataracts, and she was a diabetic too. She took her insulin and checked her sugar count many times throughout the day.

She could not have her own children and adopted all five of us, and you would never have known that we were not her own kids. She was the most unselfish, caring, and hard working mother anyone could have. She made sure that we had things even before she did.

When I was in high school she became ill, and I had to stop going to school and take care of her. My brothers and sister worked, and most of the care was on me. But, when they came home from work they were there to support me in every way. I finally did graduate from Roosevelt High School in the Bronx. What a proud day that was for everyone in my family. I became a bookkeeper and worked many jobs before getting married to my true love, Doc.

Life was great until this disease took over. I survived many operations, blood issues, and more. I had three great children and an amazing husband, who took better care of me than anyone can imagine. I miss him everyday.

I have three children who are the best in the world. I taught them responsibility and why getting an education was important. My daughter Fran always got A's in school. I was hardest on her because I knew she could handle the pressures that I put on her. She always did well in school, but if she did not get an A on a test or a perfect grade of 100 percent, I would make her write the entire test over. I felt that she needed to learn from her mistakes. She became a reading and writing specialist and worked in the NYC Public Schools. Now, she loves writing children's books, articles on many subjects, as well as this book about Alzheimer's.

My daughter Marcia attended Nancy Taylor Business School and worked for ABC News, Xerox Corporation, and now for orthopedic surgeons as their office manager. She has two great children and a lot of grandchildren. She works twelve-hour days and helps many people.

My son, Keith, has three boys and he lives in New Jersey. He tries to come and see me, but it is hard having to work over fifty hours a week and support a family.

I worked as a full charge bookkeeper for Retail Communications, Master Eagle, and Altman Electronics. I worked in many places when I was younger. I even helped out in my husband's cleaning store on 225th and Laconia Avenue, as did my girls when they were growing up.

I had many friends in my building. One friend that I miss the most is my friend Mary Kaufman. She was like a second sister to me. My daughters and my son loved her like an aunt. When my daughter Marcia would get in trouble she would run away to her apartment one flight up.

There are so many good memories in that building. I had a friend Flo whose son was my son's best friend. I have a friend Sylvia and another Shirley, who no longer live here. There are many people that are still here, but they never visit me even though they might live next door or in the same building. I guess they can't handle what has happened to me. I bet they are afraid that it will happen to them. You never know!

I had four brothers and a sister who are no longer here. I had many sisters in law that is no longer here. I have a sister-in-law named Lily who is still here, and I know she calls my children to keep in touch with how I am doing. They even call her to make sure that she is okay too.

MORE ON RUTH'S EARLY YEARS FROM FRAN

As you know from her description of herself, Ruthie was the youngest of five children. My mom never knew that her real mother died, nor did she know that during the first three months of her life her father decided to remarry since taking care of five children and working to support them would be too difficult.

Tova, my mother's oldest sibling, rebelled at having a new mother, as did Irving, Harry, and Kenny at first. Once they came to know their Aunt Katie better, they realized that she was more than just a blessing in their lives; she was great mother, too.

Katie came from Poland after being in a concentration camp and undergoing some horrific experimental tests. She was smart, astute, and although she could barely read, she was perceptive. She was someone I went to for advice when I was young. She also helped me deal with my mom when things got difficult at home.

My mother, being the youngest, was spoiled in some respects. She was blonde, had the greatest blue eyes, and always wanted to be a dancer and drum majorette. She succeeded in doing both and won baton twirling contests, but never really got too far with her dancing.

Graduating from high school was not an easy feat for her, as she had to drop out several times to care for my grandmother. When she finally graduated and realized that college was not on her horizon, she attended business school and became a full charge bookkeeper. When it came to numbers and keeping the books, my mom was equal to if not better than many accountants. She used old-fashioned pens and pencils to add, subtract, and do her figures — computers and calculators were not on Ruthie's desk at home or at work.

Times were really hard and my uncles were all in the service, so it was up to my mom and my aunt to care for my grandmother, help around the house, and still have some fun.

My Aunt Tova was a genius. No, she really was! She graduated from college at sixteen and got a teaching job right away. Imagine how proud my grandparents were, and how lucky we all were that she was able to help everyone with any schoolwork they could not grasp.

Ruthie and Tova were opposites in many ways. Tova was educationally oriented and liked to take courses in school to advance, and she loved reading books. (I guess I took after her in all of these ways.) My mom loved reading romance novels, romance magazines and the newspaper, dancing, and singing. She also loved playing canasta and mah jong, but never really had many other interests. (Before being diagnosed with Alzheimer's many years later, she had managed to raise three very smart yet very different kids.)

Being the oldest— and we won't get into age, because that's when *my* memory fades and I can't remember the exact year I was born — I was expected to set the bar and the example for everyone. From the second I entered kindergarten; I knew I was in trouble. Even creating the masterpieces that I was told to design and draw in school, I had to pass not only the teacher's inspection but Ruthie's, too.

Before entering school or being allowed to leave our micro-mini apartment on Southern Boulevard in the Bronx, my sister and I had to pass Ruthie's clothing inspection. My sister was tall, thin, blonde, and really pretty. I was overweight, not so pretty, and tall for my age up until I was ten, and then somehow I forgot to grow past five feet tall. Well, I was at least four feet wide so I guess that made up for the difference. If one of us—usually me—did not pass the to-definitely-wear inspection, we were sent back to our room to change.

My sister hated to eat breakfast, and I wanted to learn her secret of getting out of eating those awful soft-boiled eggs that my mother and grandmother insisted were healthy. (They hadn't heard of cholesterol yet.) Well, Grandma would make my eggs hard-boiled, but still I would rather have had oatmeal. (This is still true today. I never eat eggs anymore, and if I do it's only the egg whites.)

After breakfast, Marcia and I went off to school and our mother followed not too long after. Ruthie was the PTA president and her presence was required on a daily basis. The good thing was that no one dared to pick on her two perfect children — and believe me we were. To get into trouble would have earned the wrath of Ruthie. We wanted to avoid that at all costs.

Growing up with my mom, we learned values. We were also told that dating was out until you graduated college. Learning to cook, though? Well, no one was allowed near Ruthie's stove, much less Grandma's. My grandmother owned the kitchen, and when we moved, my mother owned hers.

My sister loved to bake cupcakes and of course eat them. She even made puddings and could pig out without gaining weight. All I had to do was watch her making them and I would put on forty pounds.

My mom was a firm believer in not allowing anyone to have the summer off from work or responsibility. So, my sister and I had a choice: advancing in summer school or working as a camp counselor.

While I'm giving you a glimpse of my childhood, this really is not about me, my sister, or my brother. I want to illustrate what a strong and amazing woman she was before her voice and thoughts were silenced by a deadly disease.

CHAPTER TWO

Things Aren't Quite Right

Through Ruth's Eyes Before She Knew — 2003

Initially, none of us realized my mother was having problems of any kind. She, like many Alzheimer's sufferers, thought these were just the normal signs of aging.

All of a sudden I began noticing little things that weren't quite right with me. I wasn't the same person I'd been. I could not remember where I put my glasses or my car keys. I could not remember why I walked into a room or what I was looking for. I began overdosing my meds because I did not recall taking them. This proved to be dangerous and almost fatal.

If that was not bad enough, I could not remember what I had eaten for breakfast or that I was even hungry. I forgot to get my bloods tested each month, thinking I'd had them done the month before. I never remembered calling the doctor for the results, because I did not recall taking them. Worst of all was my ability to drive a car, because my independence was about to come to an abrupt halt. Everything about my life was about to change, and there was nothing that I could do to control or stop it.

All my life I was able to manage what I was going to do and where I was going. I even managed the lives of my children so well that they turned out to do and be exactly what I wanted them to be. A mother could not be more proud.

Just the other day I drove to the small diner near where I live for breakfast with my sister, Tova. We talked about different things, and then my daughter walked in and joined us. I spilled the beans at that point. I told them that I knew I had a memory problem, and things often vanished from my mind. I told them I was scared and that even driving there I'd made some bad turns and was lucky I was not stopped.

We talked about seeing a neurologist, my primary doctor, and then we played some memory games. My daughter works with students with learning difficulties and she was able to see some of the differences in my reading and math skills right away. The she tried some mental memory tests she looked up on Google. I found after taking some of them that I could not remember dates, days of the week, or even tell time.

This was to be the first of many incidents that led my sister and me to believe that something was truly wrong and needed to be addressed. As a result of this incident and several others, my mom agreed to see my aunt's neurologist and have the dreaded MRI. She barely made it through the test due to a case of claustrophobia, and demanded the test be over pretty quickly. The next step was going to the neurologist the following week. We eventually learned through a CAT scan that she'd had a mini stroke.

I saw a doctor and I answered all of his questions, but made up some really clever answers when I could not correctly respond. For example he asked, "Ruthie, what day of the week is it?"

"There are seven," I said. "You pick one!" Smart!

When he asked me what month it was, I said, "Winter… can't you see the snow?"

When the doctor asked me to tell him how many quarters in a dollar, I told them four. But, when he asked me to multiply nine times five, I asked for a calculator. Clever!

Like a drawing on a magic slate that is there one minute and then gone the next, that is what was happening to me.

HOSPITAL STAY

On the morning of August 25, 2003 I woke up in terrible pain. The pain was in my back, but I could not describe it. My understanding of what had happened was frightening, because I could not begin to explain to anyone why I was in pain or what had caused it. I became frantic and called my sister to come down, because I did not want to scare my daughter.

By the time she called 911 and they came, I was totally incoherent and could barely tell the paramedics the degree of pain that I was in or where it was located. This was the beginning of the end, as I knew it.

I was transported to the hospital. My daughter and my sister were in the ambulance with me. The emergency staff was amazing and did all that they could to try and help find out what had caused the pain.

Unfortunately, they were not exactly correct in their diagnosis. They thought that I had an aortic aneurysm, but in reality I had overdosed on my blood thinners and had a bleed out in my left shoulder that had to be addressed before it became fatal.

Because of this I could not remain in the trauma center, and instead was taken to a different hospital and put in ICU. Unfortunately, something happened between hospitals to cause my mental status to deteriorate, and no one knew what it was.

With a breathing tube down my throat, I could not express verbally how scared I was. My family was not allowed to see me, and that made me more afraid. The following morning I heard the heart surgeon, who I had never met, call my daughter to come to the hospital to sign consent for the operation. He said it was so serious she could give her consent over the phone. But, she got there in time to see me before they wheeled me into surgery and tell me that all would be okay.

It was not okay. You know how people die and have out of body experiences? Well, I had something like that. I died twice on the table and was revived because my daughter would not allow them to give up on me. I had not signed a Do Not Resuscitate paper. When I finally came out of surgery and was awake, I realized that I could not speak because of the tubes. I also did not know what had happened or why I was there.

After two weeks in the hospital I was sent home, only to return three days later with clots in my legs. At that point I was sent to rehab and the doctors decided to find out what was really causing my problems. I knew there was a problem; why didn't they?

I was in the hospital on and off the entire month for blood clots and rehab. The agency that was supposed to send a nurse to help me always forgot. I had to have another surgery, but I was awake this time. The doctor said I needed the second surgery on my leg to clean out an infection that would not go away.

When I came home this time, the doctor made sure that the agency knew to send the nurse twice a day to clean out my wound. My daughter did not take any chances this time, and went to a different health care provider and home health care agency.

2003-2004

Throughout the rest of 2003 and into the start of 2004, I was able to live alone and take care of myself. I even started to drive again. Then one day I took my daughter to the doctor and I had a rude awakening. I came to an intersection and drove past three red lights and then went down a one-way street, telling her I knew what I was doing. Two very unfriendly police officers that wanted to give me at least eight tickets for at least eight serious violations stopped me. But, by the time my daughter explained my problem and my state of confusion, we were lucky and they let me go with a warning.

When I got home that day, my daughter told me to consider not driving any more. I would not hear of it. But, a month later the same thing happened and she and my other daughter hid the two sets of keys to the car and refused to let me drive anywhere. They told me to take Access A Ride or a car service to get where I had to go if someone was not around to drive me. I was livid, but I had no choice.

In June of that year my daughter, Marcia, sold my car in order to make sure that I did not call a locksmith to make a new set of keys.

Slowly, and deliberately, the mean and terrible web weaved by dementia started to overtake my mother's mind and body. It crept in slowly, without any warning, and BAM! overtook her with venom.

CHAPTER THREE

The Diagnosis

Why Me? — 2004

After a while my mother began to get worse, so going back to the neurologist was unnecessary. At the last visit, he told me he'd done all he could do for my mother, said my family could call any time of day and he would help them with understanding the disease. He was amazing and kept his word a thousand times over and more.

I now know I have Alzheimer's disease and there is no cure. I cannot go to the bathroom alone or be alone, because I cannot remember that I even went to the bathroom or have to go. I never remember eating so I get to eat all day. Of course that could be a plus if I was a big eater before, but I wasn't.

I have four strangers that take care of me around the clock because I cannot be alone. I do not like to be alone, and as the disease progresses so does my behavior. I never used bad language as a child and would punish my children if they did. Now, I can't seem to control it at times, nor can I control my aggressive behaviors or my mood swings. It is not menopause or hot flashes; it is the disease. I even repeat myself because I cannot remember saying whatever I said in the first place.

I live at home and my daughter sees me daily to set up my meds, give them to me, and make sure that the aides are taking good care of me. She makes sure that I have plenty of food in the fridge. On Wednesdays and Fridays she walks with me and the aide to go to the stores and we buy things. On Thursdays my other daughter comes and we go out to lunch. Last week, I think someone came to see me from my family, but I don't remember whom.

None of my friends call me, and the sad part is people that live in my building who I know for over forty years never ring my bell to say hello or see how I am doing. You never know when this disease will get you or anyone in your family. They better hope that their families care about them the way mine cares about me.

My doctor wanted my children to put me in a nursing home, but my daughter, the one with power of attorney and my health proxy, would never allow it. He now says that if not for her I would not even be here. I guess that I am not living the American dream anymore. But, I would rather be on this side of the world then on the other. At least I can still see my children, and I do know who they are and my grandchildren. I might not remember their names but I know their faces. Oh yeah! Next year I might even get to go to my grandson's bar mitzvah. I really hope I live to see it.

For all of you out there that do not call your mothers and fathers to say I love you and forget all that they did for you, start remembering it and say thank you. I am so lucky that my children appreciate all that I did and never once hesitate to make sure that I am all right now.

Maybe there will be a miracle in the near future and I will be able to remember some of what I lost. If not, I hope that others will be able to benefit from whatever medical science has to offer. I hope it is soon.

Life will never be the same for me. Many say that you need to have a certain quality of life or why bother to live? I will let God decide when it is my time to leave this world, not anyone else.

RUTH FROM HER DAUGHTER FRAN'S POINT OF VIEW

As you can see from her writings, my mother's outlook on life was remarkable. Though her mind began to wander, she tried hard not to lose sight of who she was. She held on to her sense of humor and her sense of family as long as she could. Her courage took her beyond what most people could endure. I believe her zest for life kept her alive.

My mom was a force to be reckoned with. She had her own way of doing things and expected everyone to follow suit. It was not easy to measure up to her standards, but it worked for her and after a while it worked for me, too.

Don't get me wrong, my mom was really amazing, loving, and quite distinct in her views and outlook in life. She wasn't mean or difficult to live with. As long as you followed whatever Ruthie said, your life was much easier. This also allowed you to avoid her lectures and punishment of writing out what you would have done differently had you listened to her in the first place.

My mom created a schedule for me, which included my activities before and after school and on the weekends. In this way I was never without something to do. I was lucky if she remembered to schedule time for me to eat and sleep. She was tough, smart, and quite opinionated. I guess that's why I turned out the way I am.

It was really hard to see this vital and detail oriented woman lose herself to the disease. Now it was my turn to take care of her.

CHAPTER FOUR

The Uninvited Guest

Slowly Slipping Away — Late 2004-2005

How do you say goodbye when you are still here? How do you say goodbye before your thoughts, desires, and wishes disappear from your mind? What happens when all that's left of you is a human shell? Everyone invites guests to their homes for dinner, or just to talk. But, some guests overstay their welcome and others are just plain annoying. Uninvited guests can be escorted out and asked to leave, hopefully never to return. One uninvited guest made its way inside my mother's mind and refused to leave.

Sitting in my car in front of a local diner, I just sat there staring out of the window, wondering what I was supposed to do and where I was going. Looking at the keys in my hand, they seemed like a foreign object and the ignition of the car like something you put something into, but I had no idea what. It took me a while to focus and then realize what I had to do.

For weeks now I have been forgetting where I put my keys, where I was going — even the names of people that I have known for years. I just thought it was because I had pressing problems on my mind, things cluttering my thoughts, and I never realized that I was losing memory. Not realizing the gravity of the situation but being someone that liked to have a handle on everything, I decided to keep a log of these episodes, or at least try to, but not say anything to anyone.

Days would pass and I would be fine. Maybe I would forget to shut off a light, lock the door, or even pay for bread in the bakery. Maybe I would even forget where I put my eyeglasses, but not until I made one grave mistake while driving home from the doctor's office one afternoon did I realize that something might be wrong.

This is my story before I became something or someone else. Before, I could remember everything, add columns in my head, do bookkeeping for many companies, travel by bus to the city, and even drive to my son's house to take care of his three young boys. Before, I could drive to Atlantic City, pick up friends to go to a show, and chauffeur my daughter to parties and to the homes of friends. Before, I could do anything.

Now, I tend to forget, get tired easily, and often cannot remember what I started to do, no less finish it. But, on that fateful day I was driving home and decided to take a shortcut down a one way street, pass four red lights, make a U-turn in the wrong spot, and get stopped by three police cars. You might say I was surrounded. I had no idea what I had done wrong.

This one incident will stay with me until it leaves my mind completely. You see, Alzheimer's is cruel. It does not ask your permission to come into your brain, it just does. It roams around, finds its way, and destroys all of your thought processes in its own timely fashion.

I remember sitting in a diner with my daughter having breakfast and telling her that I had trouble adding and subtracting numbers. We began practicing to try and sharpen my skills. It did help for a while.

At times I would forget names of family members, so my two daughters created albums of pictures and with my help we labeled them and went over them every day. After all, if someone did come to visit it would be nice if I remembered his or her name.

Added to these incidences, the following really started to bring home what was happening. I went out for a while and forgot to lock my door. I took what little money that I had in my wallet and went down the street to buy a loaf of bread. That in itself was okay, you might say, but what I remember doing next was dangerous.

I flagged down a car that was going my way—or at least I thought the driver was headed for my building, which was just about a block from the bakery—and offered to pay the driver to take me home. You see, my legs hurt and I was having trouble walking up the huge hill in front of my building, let alone the driveway to my building's entrance.

I also forgot that the home health aide was coming. When she arrived she claimed the door was open. She went into my apartment and called my daughter, who came straight home to finding me sitting in my favorite chair. She reminded me that what I did was dangerous.

No one yelled or screamed. Everyone explained why going into a car with a stranger could have turned tragic.

In February I began feeling sick and wound up in the hospital for another surgery. I had an aneurysm in my stomach. If not for the emergency room nurse, no one would have noticed that my amylase count was up and my liver was not functioning correctly.

Then, in May of 2005 I was out with my family for Mother's Day and I began feeling weak and light-headed. I felt a pain in my back again and asked to go home. My daughter started to drive me home when my other one said, "Straight to the hospital. Obviously, her INR is off due to a new medication she was taking that did not interact well with her Coumadin."

I spent over a week in the hospital. The staff was not that great to me one night and me they left me sitting a chair in my room and did not put me back into my bed. I could hardly walk and did not really understand what was happening. I could not reach the phone to answer it and I did not remember how to dial it.

My daughter became concerned when I did not answer the phone and she called the nurse's desk to make sure that I was okay. Although they did put me back in my bed after leaving me in the chair for over five hours, they did not seem to care about me at all. They even tried to convince my daughters to put me in a nursing home They told them they would take over my care if they did not listen. Knowing my daughter, Fran, I knew that it would never happen.

She was the one they surrounded the next morning and tried to intimidate. She took out her phone and called her attorney, and explained to them that would never happen as long as she had power of attorney and was in charge of my care.

I know that ORT is waiting for my ads for their journal. It is my job to get the ads and put the entire journal together for them. Since getting sick and not being able to driving anymore, I'm not sure how I'll get this done. Well, there is only one way. I know that my daughter will not be too thrilled to get stuck running around collecting ads and money from total strangers, but we can only hope for the best. The journal has to go to the printer before the end of next week, and since being ill I have not even put the rough draft together.

I need to get the president's message and the messages from the other officers in the organization. I need to get the ads from the store owners and any city or state officials that wanted an ad in the journal. I also needed the In Memory information or any other announcements that members wanted to place in the journal.

I'm still having trouble remembering things, but I told my daughter the best way that I could what needed to be done. Instead of getting upset she took an older journal and used it as the basis for the new one. She took my notes and wrote down all of the people who had paid for the ads or memory pages, and wrote down those that were already sent in and those she needed to get.

Never doing this before she knew that she would need help, and she asked my sister, Tova, to help her. They both went around White Plains Road in the Bronx and got as many ads as they could from the store owners where they both shopped. Then, Tova called all of her contacts in the Democratic Club and those she met when we both did voter's registration and working at the poles on election day, and they both managed to get the journal together. This would be the last one that I was able to do.

Another step in my mother's descent into the depths of Alzheimer's disease is illustrated in the following excerpt from her journal.

I decided to go to the bakery to buy two loaves of bread. Standing in line, I became impatient and demanded that I be served before anyone else. I did not care that there were at least ten other people there before me. I refused to be ignored and left waiting.

I became irritable, angry, and started yelling, and demanded that they give me two loaves of bread because I was being starved at home and no one would feed me. Of course that was not true, but I felt that this might help get me served faster. Besides, for a short moment, I actually believed what I was saying.

Cold stares of disbelief, anger, and definitely strange looks, greeted my outburst. Others were mumbling under their breath thinking I was deaf and could not hear their harsh words.

"I'm all alone," I kept saying, "and I am starving. They took all of my money and refuse to feed me. They are supposed to care for me. Look at me. I need food." Realizing that I was making a scene, the owner packed up two loaves of bread and some rolls and quietly escorted me to the door, hoping that I would just disappear or go home.

Walking home, or at least I hoped in the right direction, I stopped a stranger getting into her car and asked her for a ride home. I told her my legs hurt and I really could not walk up the huge hill to my building. This was not smart as my daughter told me later that day. But, all I wanted was to get home.

While I was dealing with the bakery people and getting food, my daughter received a frantic phone call from my home health aide, who'd arrived and found the door to my apartment unlocked and opened. No one knew where I was until I sauntered in about thirty minutes later.

This made my children realize that I could not stay at home alone any more. They hired home health aides to assist me for part of the day. I could not take my meds by myself, and my daughter had to prepare them and give them to me twice a day. I could not drive anymore, but refused to allow anyone to sell my car. I hoped in the back of my mind that I would get better and start to be my old self again.

CHAPTER FIVE

Becoming the Caregiver

Because I was the primary caregiver for my mother, I had to change my lifestyle and my way of living. I retired from teaching early to free up my time so I could deal with nurses, doctors, home care agencies, and home care providers. I found it difficult to find time for myself so I could have some type of life outside of my care-giving duties. For the next seven years after my mother's diagnosis, I rarely went anywhere.

As she got much worse, rather than making her presence known in her distinct way, she would just sit and stare at the television all day. Although the aides did try, and sometimes succeeded, in taking her out in her wheelchair to get some air and possibly run into an old friend who might stop and say hello, she would often rebel and refuse to leave her chair in front of the television. That seems to be her safety net, and she is afraid of anything different.

It was really hard for me to remain calm and neutral when other family members failed to check in on mom or went away on vacation. With them out of the picture, I couldn't take a break.

This made me upset, and I often got into it with the guilty party. I would try to explain that there are times when I would like to just do something during the day, or even stay over in a hotel with my husband for the night. I couldn't' do that if I was the only available family member, because the home health aides weren't allowed to give my mom her meds. I had to give them to her twice a day.

People forget that caregivers might actually need to do other things during the day. They also need a break from the emotionally draining reality of dealing with an Alzheimer's patient.

Caregivers are people too — not just robots who give care 24-hours a day. Family members need to understand that the primary caregiver needs time to regroup and regenerate him or herself on a regular basis.

CHAPTER SIX

The Harsh Truth Sets In

The Family Begins to Face the Inevitable — 2006

Ruth Swerdloff, the once vital and intelligent woman I knew now spends her days sitting in a chair staring at the television screen and letting the world go by.

Life is different now. I never know who's coming through that door. One day it could be a fat cow, and another someone tall and thin. I hate all of them. They stare at me and I just stick out my tongue at them because I know how they feel when they see me. I do like some of these strangers because they tell me their names when they walk in, and even say, "Good morning, Ruthie." That's me.

At least I know who I am. Joyce is great and so is Joan. They are not lazy like the others who sit on their fat duffs and do nothing but wait until their shift is over. My daughter rids me of these people right away. All I have to do is give her the sign and she understands.

Joyce and Joan are my favorite people to care for me. They make great food and even remember NO SALT! They love taking me down, and we sometimes go to Dunkin Donuts for coffee and some sweet stuff. My daughter treats everyone.

My pills are crushed and my daughter gives them to me in either yogurt or ice cream twice a day. We go to the stores when we are done and my daughter buys me new outfits to wear in case I go somewhere special. I love eating, so she and my daughter, Marcia, constantly bring great meats and other dishes to my apartment so that I never have to go hungry.

Right now I am sitting in my recliner and talking to my daughter as she records my words.

At times I can't remember events, things, or people like I did even yesterday. The world seems to be fading away and getting smaller. At least my world is.

Visions of past events come into my mind but slowly fade away. At times I feel enveloped in a huge black cloud that gets larger and larger and never goes away. Other times there seems to be a thick foggy mist around my head, covering my eyes and preventing me from seeing the world as it is.

Something has overtaken my thoughts, mind, and thinking skills. But what? I have no idea. Slowly, methodically, and carefully, like a book with its chapters outlined and set in type to be published and printed, my world seems dimmer and my memory all fogged up as this entity takes hold within the recesses of my mind, ready to print out and publish my future.

A WINDOW INTO RUTH'S WORLD — 2006

My day starts when I open my eyes and find myself sleeping on my chair. I try to get up but someone stops me. I jump at the sound of the person's voice and become frightened. I cream, "Get out of my house! Why are you here?" Then, I use some profanities and keep telling them to leave. Finally, I cry so hard and so uncontrollably that I begin to shake. All the while, this person is trying to calm me down and tells me, "Ruth, everything will be okay. It's me, Joan… you know me. I love you."

Joan stands in front of me and I really don't know her name — or anyone else's for that matter — but I do know her face. Then, my day begins with taking me to the bathroom and helping me get cleaned up. I smell something and realize that I soiled my diaper, and I am not capable of changing it. I try to tell her that but it comes out like, "I know you did it, I think so too, just do it. Don't you remember?" That seems to be what I say a lot of the time. I don't know why.

After getting me cleaned up, she takes me into another place and gives me food. I have no idea what she is giving me or what you call it. I look at it and she says it is called oatmeal. It could be anything and I would not know it. She could give me dog food or worse and I would still eat it if I felt hungry.

The trouble is…. "No good!" I can't remember what else I was going to say. I started to tell her the oatmeal was no good but I could not tell her why. I just stared out into space and forgot that I was even eating anything at all. She asked me what was no good and I began shouting, "NO GOOD! NO GOOD! NO GOOD!" and threw the spoon at her.

I think she was about to say something when my daughter walked in and saw what had happened. She looked at me covered in oatmeal and the food all over the floor, then asked Joan what caused me go get so agitated. I was trying to say that the oatmeal was too hot, but I could not remember what hot meant, or that it needed some sugar because I like things sweeter.

My daughter looked at me and just smiled. I knew everything would be okay because she was there. She came to give me something that looked like a lot of things, but I don't know why I had to take them to stay alive. Some looked like candy, some looked like round things, and the rest looked like mush. She called it my medicine and said that I needed to take these things in order to be okay. I just spit them all out and yelled "NO!"

Then all of a sudden something strange that has never happened before really puts me over the edge. I started to curse and use all kinds of bad words and could not stop myself. I kept telling whoever the fat lady was that was in my house to "Get out, you fat thing, and never come back!"

She stayed calm. She just said, "Ruthie, we all love you. It will be okay."

I just glared at her in total horror and started to try and leave. "I am not staying here with you. You can't make me. I hate you!" I was ranting like a crazy lady and could not stop. All of a sudden someone else came, and both of them just looked at me and did not know whether to laugh or cry. I don't know what I did.

I went back to sleep on my chair and let them worry about what to do. When I woke up again I did not remember what had happened before, but I knew something in me had changed. I began talking funny and sounded like something out of a horror movie. I started yelling, "WOO! WOO! WOO! WOO!" and waving my arms as if I was possessed. I started smiling strangely. I heard the two of them say I sounded like I thought I was a different person trying out different voices. I had no idea what they were talking about.

I started to pretend I was dancing and said, "I want to float and fly over there with the birds. Don't you see them?" Then I said, "I want to go over there and eat and eat all of you." I could not control my words or what I was saying.

I became so out of control that Joan had to call my neighbor and my daughter to stop me from yelling and screaming. All I kept saying was, "Don't you remember? Leave me alone! Get out of here and stop trying to kill me!" I started to speak but no one knew it was me. I sounded like three different people, and they thought I was going crazy.

Throughout the day the same things happened until I got an extra dose of Risperdal to help control my outbursts and calm me down. Even the doctor did not know what to say when they called him. His words were, "That is the disease progressing. Get used to it." Get used to what? Not knowing who you are or who anyone else happens to be? I did not even know my own daughter, who was standing next to me and trying her best to stay calm for my benefit.

What happened next was earthshaking and even worse. All of a sudden the aide saw something brown and awful on the carpet when she went to help me to the table to eat something. It went down my legs and I could not control it or stop it from coming. It looked like a river of dark chocolate. She just shook her head and took me to the bathroom and did her best not to get upset.

The rug, her shoes, the carpet, and of course me were one big mess and smell. I started to cry because I knew that I did something bad. I said, "I am bad, I am sorry. Don't yell at me." Of course no one did.

When it gets dark I get scared because I can't tell the difference between day and night. I just sit in my chair and watch whatever is on that thing in front of me. Sometimes I talk to the people on that thing and start yelling at them. If I see someone on it hurting someone, I think it is really happening. If I see something I don't like, I start screaming and yelling for someone to change it.

Life has not been the same for me for the last six years. It will probably only get worse. My children told me I am going to be 81 years old on Thanksgiving Day. I don't even know what that means. All I said when they told me I was going to my son for that day is okay. Then, "I want my son. I want him now! No one else cares about me. Just him." I guess I say that because he is always working and I really never see him except when I imagine it in my dreams.

I see a lot of people in my dreams. I see my husband and my sister who are not here anymore. I see my brothers, too. I talk to myself, and sometimes I even talk to pictures on the piano and to that thing in front of me. When am I going to be myself again? When is anyone going to be able to help me? I think the answer is NEVER!

CHAPTER SEVEN

Ruth's Final Chapter

Late 2006-2011

W hile it was difficult to see my mother's condition deteriorate day by day, the family took comfort in the fact that we'd been able to keep her at home with familiar things and loving care.

Things are really getting bad. I can barely use the phone and I became totally incontinent after a week at the hospital. My daughter had to buy supplies in order to keep me clean and dry at home. When she was finally able to get me Medicaid services, no one told her that many of the supplies were covered. She, along with my other daughter, paid out thousands of dollars for supplies and for my home care. Although she was able to get me twelve hours of Medicaid home health services, both of my daughters had to pay thousands a month for the other ninety-six hours a week. This was upsetting to them and to me. Even though I've been having trouble understanding things more and more, I know that both of them are stressed out and look worried all the time.

I did not understand how costly this stuff would be. I heard numbers like 1,500 dollars a week and saw my daughters looking upset and so despondent that I wished I could take away the sadness in their eyes and bring back the smiles.

In 2006 my daughter Frani finally got VNS to agree to the split shift home health aides, I did not know what that meant, but I could see the strain and the sadness finally melt away.

2007

Unfortunately, our fight for financial assistance was not over yet. VNS tried to take away the aides in January of 2007, but fortunately I was able to talk to them and got them to keep providing services.

My sister and I worked for two years to keep our mother's home care in place and make sure that there were no changes. It was a struggle and only promised to get harder. She had many medical issues that need to be addressed on a daily basis, as well as dietary issues that had to be met. The aides had to read labels on everything she ate to make sure there were no offending ingredients. They also made physical checks to make sure no new symptoms had shown up.

By this time, she could barely speak in full sentences and her speech was often incoherent. All we could do was be there every day and hope someone would find a cure.

2008-2010

What do you do when everyone around you is talking and you have no idea what they are saying? How do you react when your family, children, and friends are around you and you have to keep you own private scorecard in your mind as to who they are, but never quite figure it out? What do you do when the world around you seems to be fading away and you cannot stop it? This is the reality for someone with Alzheimer's disease.

Quicksand will send you down a deep hole real fast and you won't know what hit you, and there is no way to pull yourself out unless you get help real fast. A tsunami runs its own course and the devastation and the havoc created is insurmountable. An earthquake strikes and you are left homeless, helpless, and injured. But, when your mind is taken over by a hidden force that slowly seeps within the crevices of your brain and takes hold of your every thought, leaving you helpless to fight even though you try, life takes on a different meaning and you begin to forget why you are still here.

I think about this as I read my mother's journal and I'm glad she made sure things were down in writing while she still could. This disease is a raging inferno that starts with a small spark and burns until your mind disintegrates and nothing is left.

2011 — RUTH'S FIGHT IS OVER

My mom stayed at home and she had four home health aides who were amazing. Her doctors did all they could do for her. There are no new treatments and no new medications approved by the FDA to help her or anyone else with this disease. She finally gave up her fight on March 7, 2011 at 9:33 a.m.

I know that there are medications being tested in foreign countries and many types of research being done, but they are not available here in the United States. I only hope that someday our government decides to really put some money and effort into curing or at least halting this disease by giving more money for Alzheimer's research. I just came from my mom's house and I wanted to tell her about my two books, and my second being showcased or spotlighted on "Author's Events" by Ernie Johnson. I did tell her and she smiled. I know that somewhere inside of her she is proud of me.

PART TWO

Tips for Caregivers and Loved Ones

CHAPTER EIGHT

Taking Care of the Caregiver

All too often, as caregivers we become so immersed in taking care of the needs of the person who is ill that we forget about our own. As the primary and only caregiver for my mom, I found that I had to develop different ways to keep myself active and my mind stimulated. When you make the decision to care for the family member at home, you are taking on a challenge of Herculean proportion. Every day brings different challenges that must be handled with kindness and care.

The following tips will help you to keep things in perspective and avoid becoming burned out by the huge responsibility:

- **Remember to make time for yourself and your family.** Do not neglect your personal appearance or your personal needs. Make sure that you take time for yourself every day. You should develop an interest or a hobby and set aside time, as I do, to pursue what makes you happy.

- **Make sure to take a break when you feel stressed.** Go out for a walk, rest, or just read a book. You cannot be on twenty-four hours a day. If the person in your care needs an aide, make sure that you get the services needed in order to help you have some kind of life and time with your family.

- **Being the primary caregiver.** I know that there is always one person in a family who gets the main burden. That, of course, is not exactly fair, but it is what it is. If this is your role, you need to make sure that you get to go away, even overnight or on a weekend, to rejuvenate yourself and feel better. You deserve it. I know I needed time off from giving my mom her meds every morning and every night. I sometimes felt like I was wearing a straight jacket that needed to be loosened. I wished I could go away for a week, but I knew that was not in the cards. No one wants the responsibility of dealing with the agencies and the meds and the aides — it's tough. I was told so many times, "You're doing the right thing, and someday you'll be blessed and rewarded for it." What I know is that I can look myself in the eye and know I have nothing to feel guilty about, I did my best and kept my mother at home as she wished. If you are the primary caregiver, be sure to take care of yourself, too.

CHAPTER NINE

Tips for Caregivers

DISCUSSIONS AND TALKING

When a person has Alzheimer's the hardest thing to deal with is their forever changing and erratic behaviors. The person can be calm one minute and then out of control or violent the next. These behaviors put a lot of stress on the caregiver. Here are some things that worked with my mom that might help when dealing with these radical mood changes:

- Speaking slowly and softly to calm the person down.

- Speaking in simple sentences and short phrases.

- Repeating something in different ways to help with understanding what she needs to do. For example, when trying to feed him or her, say, "Open your mouth," rather than becoming frustrated and trying to explain why he or she needs to eat.

- Calling them by their first name, or of course Mom, to get their attention.

- Be positive and smile at the person. Do not let them think you are angry or disappointed.

BATHING

- **Create a daily schedule.** Knowing what to expect can be comforting for the person and help to keep things on track for the caregiver.

- **Gentle touch.** Always be kind and gentle when bathing the person, and always pick out clothing that is easy to put on and take off.

- **Explanations.** Explain what you are going to do and why, even if the person does not fully understand.

- **Prepare beforehand.** Collect soap, sponges, etc. and have the shower head ready before the bathing begins.

- **Be safe.** Be sure the person is seated either on a bench in the tub or on a shower chair to prevent falls. If a handheld shower head, is not available then a sponge bath might be the next best option.

GETTING DRESSED

- Create a schedule. Again, having a scheduled time for getting dressed each day and having hair and nails done can be helpful with making the person feel like they are still a part of life. Making things as normal as possible can go a long way.

- Store some clothes in another room to reduce the number of choices. Keep only one or two outfits in the closet or dresser.

- Choose clothing that is comfortable, easy to get on and off, and easy to care for. Elastic waists and Velcro® enclosures minimize struggles with buttons and zippers, and slip on shoes are easy.

- Arrange the clothes in the order they are to be put on to help the person move through the process.

- Allow the person to choose from a limited selection of outfits. If he or she has a favorite outfit, consider buying several identical sets. Doing this will make them feel like they still have control over at least one part of their lives during a time when everything else is out of control for them.

- Encourage the person to dress him or herself or herself to whatever degree possible. Plan to allow extra time so there is no pressure or rush.

- Hand the person one item at a time or give clear, step-by-step instructions if the person needs prompting.

MEAL TIME

Encouraging someone with Alzheimer's to eat can be a real challenge especially in the late stages of the illness. Here are some tips to make things easier for both the person and the caregivers:

- View mealtimes as opportunities for social interaction and success for the person with Alzheimer's. Try to be patient and avoid rushing, and be sensitive to confusion and anxiety.

- Aim for a quiet, calm, reassuring mealtime atmosphere by limiting noise and other distractions.

- Maintain familiar mealtime routines, but adapt to the person's changing needs.

- Give the person food choices, but limit the number of choices. Try to offer appealing foods that have familiar flavors, varied textures, and different colors.

- Serve small portions or several small meals throughout the day. Make healthy snacks, finger foods, and shakes available. In the earlier stages of dementia, be aware of the possibility of overeating.

- Choose dishes and eating tools that promote independence. If the person has trouble using utensils, use a bowl instead of a plate, or offer utensils with large or built-up handles. Use straws or cups with lids to make drinking easier.

- Encourage the person to drink plenty of fluids throughout the day to avoid dehydration.

- As the disease progresses, be aware of the increased risk of choking because of chewing and swallowing problems.

- Maintain routine dental checkups and daily oral health care to keep the mouth and teeth healthy.

ACTIVITIES

Finding activities that the person with Alzheimer's disease can do and is interested in can be a challenge. Building on current skills generally works better than trying to teach something new.

- Don't expect too much. Simple activities often are best, especially when they use current abilities.

- Help the person get started on an activity. Break the activity down into small steps and praise the person for each step he or she completes.

- Watch for signs of agitation or frustration with an activity. Gently help or distract the person to something else.

- Incorporate activities the person seems to enjoy into your daily routine and try to do them at a similar time each day.

- Try to include the person with Alzheimer's in the entire activity process. For instance, at mealtimes, encourage the person to help prepare the food, set the table, pull out the chairs, or put away the dishes. This can help maintain functional skills, enhance feelings of personal control, and make good use of time.

- Take advantage of adult day services, which provide various activities for the person with Alzheimer's, as well as an opportunity for caregivers to gain temporary relief from tasks associated with care-giving. Transportation and meals often are provided.

INCONTINENCE

- **Supplies.** You may not have to pay for supplies, including diapers, ointments and salves out of pocket. Medicaid and Hospice are two sources to check.

- **Create a schedule.** Set up a bathroom or changing schedule for the person to prevent rashes, sores and chafing. The aides change my mom every two hours to prevent rashes, sores, and chafing.

- **Visual clues.** If the person fidgets or acts restless, this can be a sign they need the bathroom, if they are still capable.

- **Keep calm.** Be aware that accidents will happen and you need to stay calm and be understanding. The person wants to remain diaper free and independent for as long as possible, so accidents will be upsetting to them because this is a signal that this independence is coming to an end.

- **Limit evening fluids.** To prevent nighttime accidents, limit the amount of fluids containing caffeine in the evening.

- **Field trips.** If the person is able to travel outside the home, be sure to plan for frequent stops and bring along extra clothing and incontinence supplies.

SAFETY PRECAUTIONS

- **Safe Return.** It is a good idea to enroll the person in the Safe Return Program from the Alzheimer's Association (there is a cost for this service). If a registered individual with Alzheimer's or a related dementia wanders and becomes lost, caregivers can call the 24-hour emergency response line to report it. A community support network will be activated, including local Alzheimer Association chapters and law enforcement agencies, to help reunite the person with the caregiver or a family member. With this service, critical medical information will also be provided to emergency responders when needed.

- **Photograph.** Keep a photo of the person in your wallet, in your living room, and in their home in case the person is lost and ID needs to be made by the police.

- **Medications.** Keep a list of the person's medications and other vital information handy, including dosages. Post this info on the refrigerator along with their plan of care if you have home care, and keep a copy with you in your phone, tablet or wallet.

- Install secure locks on all outside windows and doors, especially if the person is prone to wandering. Remove the locks on bathroom doors to prevent the person from accidentally locking himself or herself in.

- Use childproof latches on kitchen cabinets and anyplace where cleaning supplies or other chemicals are kept.

- Label medications and keep them locked up. Also make sure knives, lighters and matches, and guns are secured and out of reach.

- Keep the house free from clutter. Remove throw rugs and anything else that might contribute to a fall.

- Make sure lighting is good both inside and outside the home.

- Be alert to and address kitchen-safety issues, such as the person forgetting to turn off the stove after cooking. Consider installing an automatic shut-off switch on the stove to prevent burns or fire.

VISITS, FAMILY GATHERINGS AND HOLIDAYS

- For the holidays, keep or adapt family traditions that are important to you. Include the person with Alzheimer's as much as possible.

- Recognize that things will be different, and be realistic about what you can do.

- Encourage friends and family to visit. Limit the number of visitors at one time, and try to schedule visits during the time of day when the person is at his or her best.

- Avoid crowds, changes in routine, and strange places that may cause confusion or agitation.

- At larger gatherings such as weddings or family reunions, try to have a space available where the person can rest, be alone, or spend some time with a smaller number of people, if needed.

COMMUNICATING WITH RESPECT AND KINDNESS

- SMILE!

- Be calm and quiet. Avoid using a loud tone of voice or talking to the person as if he or she were a child.• When you speak, make eye contact.

- Speak clearly.

- Use simple and direct statements.

- Never raise your voice.

- Include the person in your conversation. Talk to the person, not at the person.

- Never speak as if they are a third party, and do not discuss them with someone else if they're in the same room.

- Listen to their concerns and show a lot of understanding.

- Respect the person's personal space and don't get too close.

- Remind the person who you are if he or she doesn't seem to recognize you.

- Don't argue if the person is confused. Respond to the feelings you hear being communicated, and distract the person to a different topic if necessary.

- Remember not to take it personally if the person doesn't recognize you, is unkind, or responds angrily. He or she is reacting out of confusion.

CHAPTER TEN

How Do You Know When Your Loved One Needs Help?

W hen people with dementia no longer understand their own safety and can't look after themselves, family members and health-care professionals may need to weigh the risks of living alone against the benefits of supporting him or her to live at home. In many families, care-giving falls to one person. Hold a family meeting when he or she is at an early stage of the disease, so that you can plan what each family member can realistically do to help, now and in the future.

People with Alzheimer's disease need to live in safe environments that support quality of life. The amount and type of support available are important factors in determining if a person can live alone. For example, a person with a large family, or someone who lives in a community with many services may be better able to live alone than someone with no family, living in a community with limited services.

Family members and health-care professionals can help reduce risks for people with dementia who want to live alone. For example, if he frequently leaves the stove on, consider disconnecting the stove and finding other ways to provide hot food, such as Meals on Wheels.

Wherever possible, the person with the disease should take part in discussions concerning their own future.

Here are some factors to consider:

OVERALL WELL-BEING

- What is his/her quality of life at home?

- Is there a good balance of stimulation during the day?

- Could he/she benefit from the level of care and support provided by another environment, such as a son or daughter's home, retirement home or long-term care home?

- Is there help from community support agencies?

HEALTH

- Is he/she able to take medication properly?

- If sick, would he/she be able to understand and take appropriate action, such as calling for help?

- Is he/she able to take care of personal hygiene, such as bathing and toileting?

- Are there current or past health problems that might put him/her at risk of harm?

NUTRITION

- Is he/she able to maintain a proper weight?

- Is he/she able to eat nutritiously throughout the day?

- Is he/she able to store and prepare foods properly?

- Is he/she eating inappropriately (cat food)?

SAFETY

- Is he/she at risk of harm? If yes, is the amount of risk acceptable to her? To family members? To caregivers?

- Is it possible to find a level of risk with which everyone is comfortable? For example, the risk of falling on the stairs might be considered an acceptable risk if he/she has no problems with balance or walking.

- Does the he/she pose a risk to others? For example, does she live in an apartment and cause fires with the stove or cigarettes?

- Is he/she able to react and take appropriate action in an emergency, such as a fire?
- Is his/her home safe? For example, are stairs well lit? Are there handrails?
- Do individuals or organizations check in with him/her regularly and in the event of a blackout or other emergency situations?

FINANCES

- Can he/she handle day-to-day financial transactions, such as keeping track of bills and paying bills promptly?
- Is he/she at risk of exploitation or abuse regarding finances?
- Can he/she handle day-to-day financial transactions, such as keeping track of bills and paying bills promptly?

FINDING THE RIGHT CARE

It is hard to decide what the right kind of care is for the person. It is hard at times to convince an independent person that they are going to require this care and that the illness is what will determine the care and how fast it progresses.

The following tasks will require some help and eventually, as with my mom, permanent help.

- Shopping
- Paying bills
- House cleaning
- Meals
- Using the phone
- Laundry
- Transportation

YOU MAY NEED HELP WITH THESE TOO:

- Bathing and getting dressed
- Toileting

- Getting in and out of chairs, beds

- Eating and taking medications

TYPES OF CARE

There are a number of different types of care to consider when deciding what your loved one needs.

IN HOME CARE

- **Companion services:** help with supervision, recreational activities, and visiting

- **Personal care services:** help with bathing, dressing, toileting, exercising, and other daily activities.

- **Homemaker services:** help with housekeeping, shopping, and meal preparation

- **Home health care ordered by a physician**: provided by a licensed health worker.

ADULT DAY CENTER

- Adult day services: supervision of activities in a structured setting

- Adult day health services: supervision of activities and basic health needs in a structured setting

RESIDENTIAL CARE

- **Independent Living:** Some people find it difficult to live alone and need assistance of some kind. A private residence within a community of seniors without the need of personal or medical care can be provided.
- **Board and Care:** Group residence that provides personal and supportive services is often another option.
- **Assisted Living:** Staff monitored residence that provides personal and supportive services
- **Continuing care retirement community:** This has varying levels of care based on a person's individual needs.

- **Nursing Home:** Full range of care; offers both short-and long term care

ACUTE CARE REHABILITATION

Is short-term care offered for people with injuries, illnesses, or post-operative care needs who will eventually be able to recover in an environment outside a hospital.

LONG-TERM CARE

Is provided to individuals who require longer stays. Medicare may pay for some nursing home care, but only if you meet certain qualifications and conditions.

A nursing home is not a hospital. In a home most of the residents eat in a dining room. And, an activity director may plan activities for and with the residents.

Every home is different and unique. Different homes have different staff-to-resident ratios, and the staff at one home may be more experienced with dementia than the staff at another. You need to do your research and find out about a home before choosing that one for yourself or a loved one. You need to find out their rating and the amount of complaints that may have been filed against the home to make sure that you or a loved one are in a safe environment.

INFORMAL CARE

Many times, a family member, friend, neighbor, or even a volunteer is willing to help with the care-giving duties, giving the caregiver time to run errands or take a break or a deep breath. Caregivers should keep in mind people who have offered to help.

EMERGENCY CARE

Accidents and surgeries or unexpected trips to the hospital can create a need for care in an emergency room. In case this does happen, it is helpful to have done research and planning ahead of time about you where you can turn for this type of care.

Sources include the National Institute on Aging and www.medicinenet.com.

CHAPTER ELEVEN

Understanding and Dealing with All of the Changes

The mild and beginning stages of Alzheimer's disease dementia will bring changes in the overall functioning of the person. In order to be a caregiver you need to understand how to manage stress and be healthier. Here are ten ways to do that:

1. Understand what is going on with your loved one as early as possible.

2. Discover what resources are available in your community.

3. Become an educated caregiver.

4. Get help…seek out the support of family, friends, and community resources. Know that there is a 24/7 hot line that you can call at 1-800-272-3900. There are online message boards and local support groups that you can join.

5. Take care of YOURSELF! Watch your diet, exercise, and eat right. Get plenty of rest and keep all of your medical appointments. If you get sick it will not help the person you are taking care of.

7. Manage your level of stress.

8. Accept changes as they happen.

9. Make legal and financial plans.

10. Give yourself credit, not guilt.

11. Visit your doctor regularly.

KEEPING THINGS RUNNING SMOOTHLY

It is hard to be the sole caregiver of a person who has this disease. I know how difficult it is because of my mom and all that I go through helping her and working with her aides on a daily basis. So, for all of you wonderful, giving, and caring people who give up part of their lives or more to take care of a parent, child, or grandparent afflicted with ALZ, these tips are for you and I want you to know that you are not alone… you are truly special!

CREATING A SAFE SETTING

- **Eliminate clutter, noise, glare, and too much background noise.** I noticed with my mom that when anyone yelled or talked too loudly or constantly, it bothered her. She would put her hands over her ears or just tune someone out if they were babbling on and on.

- **Develop soothing rituals with regular daily routines, comforting objects, gentle music, and a reassuring touch.** My mom loved to watch "Dancing with the Stars" and "American Idol." She loved to watch ice-skating and programs with music and dancing and old movies on TCM, even though she really didn't understand the plot anymore. But, when she saw Fred Astaire or Ginger Rogers dance, or heard Debbie Reynolds or Gene Kelly sing she would clap her hands and smile. She did not like programs that had people yelling and screaming at each other. When the aides watched a judge program and the discussions got heated, she tended to get upset and react badly in her own special way.

- **Provide opportunities for exercise and satisfying activities geared to the person's abilities.** Before my mom went into the last stages of Alzheimer's, she loved to go to the stores to shop, even when she was in a wheelchair. She also enjoyed going to luncheons with friends from her organizations that she ran before getting sick. She loved to sit downstairs with friends and talk..

- **Monitor personal comfort and ensure a comfortable temperature, and check regularly for pain, hunger, thirst, constipation, full bladder, fatigue, infection, and skin irritation.** After a while my mom did not know whether something hurt her or not. She often expressed that she was hungry but she really wasn't. She had problems expressing herself. When it came time to eat, she would often push away the food or spit it out.

- **One of the most difficult things for an Alzheimer's patient is to expressing themselves so others can understand what they are trying to convey.** Be sensitive and understanding of frustration about expressing wants and needs. You might have to show the person what you think they want or answer the question for them. My mother reached the point where it was difficult to tell what she wanted or needed. She refused medication at times and would not eat or drink. The aides were trained and more experienced than me, so they knew how to coax her to eat and drink.

- **Do not argue with the person; redirect their attention to something else that would prevent them from getting upset or frustrated.**

- **Simplify the tasks and routines.**

- **Avoid asking open-ended questions.** Try questions that require only a yes or no answer. Of course, in the later stages of the illness this becomes more difficult.

- **Allow the person to rest between stimulating events, such as visits from friends and neighbors.** The problem with friends and neighbors is that they forget the person is there and would benefit greatly from a visit. Visits stimulate the person's mind and help to keep them more mentally active. I know that even though my mom didn't communicate verbally in a coherent way, when she saw old friends on the street or sitting on the benches, she smiled. She might not know their names, but sometimes their faces seem familiar to her in her own way.

- **Use labels to cue or remind the person.** When my mom was first diagnosed with the illness it was suggested that we label the rooms and the objects in them so that she could read what they were and hopefully remember the things in her house. I would show her pictures of the family and have the name of the person written under it so she could read it and know the family member or friend whose picture she was looking at.

- **Equip doors and gates with safety locks.**

- **Remove any weapons: guns or anything dangerous.**

PLANNING FOR THE FUTURE

Asking for help is not easy. Knowing when to make changes to the care of a person with this disease is difficult. Providing good care means meeting the needs of the person that is receiving it and planning ahead for the person's future.

As a caregiver, it became quite apparent that my mom needed help beginning in 2004, and then more serious help and care the following year, and of course in the present.

We started with four hours a day paid for care for the first six months. After my mom spent a week in the hospital and had many visits to the ER, my sister and I realized that her home care needed to be increased and that we would now have to figure out how to get that care even if we had to pay for it at first.

We were not able to get Medicaid that first year, and we wound up paying thousands of dollars for my mom's care, putting both my sister and me in debt. But, we had made the decision to never put her in nursing home, a promise we had made to our mom before her decision making skills were no longer there.

How much care a person will need depends on how independently he or she can walk, eat, use the bathroom, and bathe. As the disease progresses the person can no longer do any of these things without help.

These are the questions that you need to answer when considering more care:

- **Safety:** Is the person with dementia safe and able to stay alone?

- **Health:** Is the health of the person with dementia or the health of the caregiver at risk?

- **Care Needs:** Does the person with dementia need more care than he or she is receiving right now? Is caring for the person becoming more difficult for the primary care provider?

MOST IMPORTANT AND FINAL NOTES

- Remember to be sensitive to the needs of the person.

- Understand that the diagnosis is upsetting and show compassion.

- Remember to speak to the person as an adult and a human being and not a small child.

- Communicate with the Alzheimer's patient.

- Have an upbeat and positive attitude.

- Understand and learn how to handle behavior changes.

- Expect that the patient will have memory loss, and over time it will even get worse.

- Get support for yourself and make sure that you do not neglect you.

- Speak in short, familiar words, phrases and simple sentences. Repeat yourself if necessary. Stay calm.

- Allow the person plenty of time to answer. If the person does not respond or answer reword the question.

- Ask only one question at a time.

- Never give negative instructions. Do not say, "Don't" or "Never" or "You'd better not." Say, "Let's try this" or "Let's go over here."

- Shopping can help them stay focused and feeling useful!

- Your visit and care makes all the difference!

- Helping someone with a smile makes a difference in the other person's life.

- Remember: Everything you do matters and is special.

CAREGIVERS ARE SPECIAL AND UNIQUE!

THE PARTNERSHIP BETWEEN YOU AND YOUR LOVED ONE

The roles of many children change when a parent or grandparent is diagnosed with the illness. We accept this person until Alzheimer's disease overtakes them and changes them drastically. With this condition certain changes in roles and relationships are to be expected. People who were once independent and able to care for themselves may have to accept help for the first time in his or her life. A child may have to support the parent who has always supported him or her. These adjustments are difficult to make at the beginning. You need to understand that it will benefit everyone if you keep this in mind as a partnership in order for the person to maintain some kind of control and dignity.

This changing relationship between you and the person with the disease is similar to those who play sports and rely on another play for backup or to lead them to a winning victory. The caregiver may have to do a little more leading and less following. You need to be flexible in order for this to work.

Resources used:

www.alz.org
www.nia.nih.gov
www.nia.nih.gov/Alzheimers
www.nia.nih.gov/Alzheimers/Publications/caregiverguide.htm#intro
www.nia.nih.gov/Healthinformation/Publications/forgetfulness.htm

CHAPTER TWELVE

The Caregiver's Role is Important and Valuable

The job of caregiver is special and important. Never think that because you are not getting paid to be a volunteer that it hinders your value, importance, or role. Many of the people you come in contact with have no family members visiting, are afraid to be alone, and might look forward to your visit, no matter how long or short, as the highlight of their day.

Just walking into their room and them knowing that you are there to speak to them, perform a needed task, or just to sit and talk with them can be the difference between someone giving up on life and feeling needed and special.

Everything you do has value and a purpose. Never allow anyone to tell you that you do not have be at work or volunteer on a specific day because it does not matter since you are not getting paid. Work ethics need to be adhered to. Volunteer positions can lead to paying ones. You never know. Your time is valuable and what you are doing to help someone that is in these facilities is worth more than all the money in the world. Never underestimate the importance of what you're doing.

- Seek support from other caregivers. You are not alone!

- Take care of your own health so that you can be strong enough to take care of your loved one.

- Accept offers of help and suggest specific things people can do to help you.

- Learn how to communicate effectively with doctors.

- Caregiving is hard work so take respite breaks often.

- Watch out for signs of depression and don't delay in getting professional help when you need it.

- Be open to new technologies that can help you care for your loved one.

- Organize medical information so it's up to date and easy to find.

- Make sure legal documents are in order.

- Give yourself credit for doing the best you can in one of the toughest jobs there is!

CAREGIVER ORGANIZATIONS, INFORMATION, ADVOCACY AND SUPPORT RESOURCES

- **Caregiver Action Network:** http://www.caregiveraction.org

- **Lots a Helping Hands**
  Are you a caregiver juggling care for a loved one while keeping up with the responsibilities of everyday life? Or do you know someone caring for others and find yourself wondering how you can help? At Lotsa, we believe it takes a Community to support the caregiver. Care-giving is an extra job that few are prepared for. Our Help Calendar and community building features make it easy to organize help for the people you care about.
  Website: www.lotsahelpinghands.com

- **Children of Aging Parents (CAPS)**
  CAPS assists caregivers of the elderly with information and referrals, a network of support groups, and publications and programs that promote public awareness of the value and the needs of family caregivers.
  Phone: 800-227-7294. Website: www.caps4caregivers.org

- **Family Caregiver Alliance (FCA)**
  FCA is the lead agency in California's system of Caregiver Resource Centers. FCA provides support and help to family caregivers and champions their cause through education, services, research and advocacy. Services are specific to California, although information can be accessed nationally.
  Phone: 800-445-8106. Website: http://www.caregiver.org

- **Family Voices, Inc.**
  Family Voices offers information on healthcare policies relevant to special needs children in every state.
  Phone: 888-835-5669. Website: www.familyvoices.org

- **Friends' Health Connection**
  Friends' Health Connection links persons with illness or disability and their family caregivers with others experiencing the same challenges.
  Phone: 800-483-7436. Website: www.48friend.org

- **National Alliance for Caregiving**
  Although not an organization that helps family care-givers directly, The National Alliance for Caregiving's Website helps family caregivers learn about information, videos, pamphlets, etc. that have been reviewed and approved as providing solid information.
  Website: www.caregiving.org

- **National Family Caregivers Association**
  CAN is a national nonprofit organization dedicated to empowering family caregivers to act on behalf of themselves and their loved ones, and to remove barriers to their health and wellbeing. CAN concentrates its efforts in three primary areas: education, building community, and advocacy. For more information visit: www.thefamilycaregiver.org.
  Phone: 800-896-3650. Website: www.thefamilycaregiver.org

- **Rosalynn Carter Institute for Human Development (RCI)**
  RCI provides educational programs for caregivers, conducts research, and disseminates information about care-giving.

  Phone: 229-928-1234. Website: www.rci.gsw.edu

- **U.S. Department of Health and Human Services**
  A federal Web site designed to help people stay healthy. Healthfinder.gov features links to more than 6,000 government and nonprofit health information resources on hundreds of health topics including personalized health tools such as health calculators, activity and menu planners, recipes, and online checkups. In addition, the site offers tips for caregivers and health news. Information is provided in English and Spanish.

  Website: www.healthfinder.gov

- **Well Spouse Association**
  Well Spouse is a national membership organization that gives support to husbands, wives and partners of the chronically ill and/or disabled. Well Spouse has a network of support groups and also a newsletter for spouses.

  Phone: 800-838-0879. Website: www.wellspouse.org

CAREGIVERS AND HOME HEALTH AIDES

Home health aides and caregivers have the same jobs and must be considered equals. I know that without the knowledge and help of my mom's aides I couldn't have made it through her illness. I would have had no life outside of taking care of her daily needs, giving her the meds twice a day and staying with her around the clock. These people became a part of my family and I appreciated all that they did. Words alone cannot tell you how grateful we were that we had each of these kind, understanding, and compassionate people to care for our mom.

The following is a letter I wrote to the agency that helped to care for my mother. I wanted to show exactly how we felt about the aides who helped so much.

May 28, 2008

Partners In Care
1250 Broadway
New York, New York 10001
Attention: Veronica Collins

Dear Veronica:

There are people that you meet in life that touch your heart and make more than a lasting impression when they say hello. From the time my family and I met Joan Glover and Patricia Rich we knew that we had not only two of the best and most professionally qualified home health aides in the business, but two new family members as well. Both Joan and Pat have gone above and beyond to help take care of our mom. Our mom has Alzheimer's, and it takes a special person to understand the disease and care for a person that has it. Not only do they both take superior care of our mom, but also they have taught us all how to cope with her behaviors and how to handle the things that she says and does on a daily basis.

For the past several months both Joan and Pat have worked overtime to make sure that our mom does not have to deal with strangers during the absence of Lahoma Dennis. Our mom finds it difficult to understand and deal with someone that is new, and finds herself getting frustrated when trying to express her feelings. She can become difficult to handle and often says things that a new person might not understand or want to if not properly trained. Without Joan and Pat I do not know if I would be able to cope with the many things that I see happening to our mom each day. She needs the consistency in her life. She does not trust strangers, and although Laurel and Sarah are quite good with her, she still becomes agitated when she does not see her Joan and her Pat. Please don't forget that on Sunday, Monday and Tuesday Joyce is with her during the day, and she is amazing as well. I really feel that both Joan and Pat need to be recognized in a special way for their kindness, caring, and exemplary way of caring for our mom.

Please note that without the help of their supervisor, Veronica Collins, none of this would have been possible. Since Veronica has been her case manager, everything and every change has gone smoothly and with no aggravation. I hope that you will recognize her as well.

Thank you from my family to your family at Partners In Care. I do not know what we would do without you, and hope we never will.

Sincerely,
Fran Lewis and the family of Ruth Swerdloff

PART THREE

Resources

CHAPTER THIRTEEN

Resources and Information from the Alzheimer's Association

The Alzheimer's Association has developed the following list of warning signs that include common symptoms of Alzheimer's disease. Individuals who exhibit several of these symptoms would see a physician for a complete evaluation:

1. Memory loss

2. Difficulty performing familiar tasks

3. Problems with language

4. Disorientation to time and place

5. Poor or decreased judgment

6. Problems with abstract thinking

7. Misplacing things

8. Changes in mood or behavior

9. Changes in personality

10. Loss of initiative

It is normal for certain kinds of memory, such as the ability to remember lists of words, to decline with normal aging. In fact, normal individuals fifty years of age will recall only about 60% as much on some kinds of memory tests as individuals twenty years of age. Every twenty year old is well aware of multiple times he or she could not think of an answer on a test that he or she once knew. But, most twenty year olds do not worry about forgetting something, or that he or she has the early stages of Alzheimer's. But, a person fifty or sixty years of age with a few memory lapses may worry that they have the early stages of the disease.

BASICS OF ALZHEIMER'S DISEASE: WHAT IS IT AND WHAT CAN YOU DO

Many of us notice slowed or delayed thinking, or that we have difficulty remembering things. However, serious memory loss, confusion, and other major changes in the way our minds work are not a normal part of aging.

There are many conditions that disrupt memory and mental function. These symptoms may improve when the underlying cause is treated.

Possible reasons or causes for memory loss:

- Depression
- Medication side effects
- Excess use of alcohol
- Thyroid problems
- Poor diet
- Vitamin deficiencies
- Certain infections
- Alzheimer's disease and related dementia

ALZHEIMER'S DISEASE VS. NORMAL MEMORY CHANGES

ALZHEIMER'S SUFFERER	AGE-RELATED CHANGES
Forgets whole experiences	Forgets part of an experience
Rarely remembers those experiences later	Often remembers those experiences later
Is gradually unable to follow written/spoken directions	Is usually able to follow written/spoken directions
Is gradually unable to use notes	Is usually able to use notes
Is gradually unable to care for self	Is usually able to care for self

If you experience significant memory problems you need to see a doctor. Early diagnosis and intervention methods are improving, and treatment options and sources of support can improve your quality of life.

TEN SIGNS OF ALZHEIMER'S DISEASE

1. **Memory loss:** You forget recently learned information. This is a most common early sign of dementia. You begin to forget more often and are unable to recall information later.

2. **Difficulty performing familiar tasks:** People with dementia often find it hard to plan or finish everyday tasks. These people may lose track of the steps involved in preparing a meal, placing a phone call, or playing a game.

3. **Problems with language:** People with Alzheimer's disease often forget simple words or substitute unusual words, making their speech or writing hard to understand. They may be unable to find the toothbrush, and may ask for that thing for my mouth instead.

4. **Disorientation to time and place:** People with this disease can become lost in their own neighborhoods, forget where they are and how they got there, and not know how to get back home.

5. **Poor or decreased judgment:** People with the disease often dress inappropriately, wearing many layers on a warm day and/or little clothing in the cold. They may show poor judgment

about money by giving away large amounts to telemarketers over the phone.

6. **Problems with abstract thinking:** Some with Alzheimer's disease may have unusual trouble performing complex mental tasks, like forgetting what numbers are and how they should be used.

7. **Misplacing things:** A person with this disease may put things in unusual places. This person might put an iron in the freezer or a wristwatch in the refrigerator.

8. **Changes in mood or behavior:** Someone with this disease may show rapid mood swings—from calm to tears to anger—for no apparent reason.

9. **Changes in Personality:** The personalities of people with dementia can change dramatically. They may become extremely confused, suspicious, fearful, or dependent on a family member.

10. **Loss of initiative:** A person with this disease may become very passive, sitting in front of the TV for hours, sleeping more than usual or not wanting to do usual activities.

NORMAL MEMORY LAPSES

1. Forgetting names or appointments occasionally.

2. Occasionally forgetting why you came into a room or what you planned to do.

3. Sometimes having trouble finding the right word.

4. Forgetting the day of the week or where you were going.

5. Making questionable or debatable decisions from time to time.

6. Challenging to balance a checkbook.

7. Misplacing keys or a wallet temporarily.

8. Occasionally feeling sad or moody.

9. People's personalities do change somewhat with age.

10. Sometimes feeling weary of work or social obligations.

Doctor Discussion Guide

When your family member is concerned about the changes mentioned in the previous section that might indicate mild to moderate Alzheimer's disease of dementia.

The following information comes from the website of Novartis. These are the questions that you need to ask your doctor:

1. Do the symptoms indicate a problem?

2. Is Alzheimer's disease dementia one of the possible things that might be causing these symptoms?

3. Are there other conditions that might be causing these symptoms?

4. Will tests be needed in order for you to make this diagnosis? Which ones?

5. How long will it be before I will know the diagnosis?

6. If it is Alzheimer's disease, what should I expect?

7. What medicines are available?

8. Can these medicines help slow the worsening of symptoms? Which ones?

9. How do these medicines work?

QUESTIONS YOUR DOCTOR MIGHT ASK YOU OR A FAMILY MEMBER
1. Are you or someone you care for:
   a. Forgetting conversations, appointments, or holidays?

   b. Having difficulty finding the right words to express their thoughts or your thoughts?

   c. Repeating stories or questions?

   d. Getting lost in places familiar to you/them?

2. Have you or someone you care for:
   a. Forgotten how to do familiar activities, like cooking or repairing things?

b. Had difficulty doing bills or balancing the checkbook, or thrown away a bill before paying it?

c. Been misplacing things more often than usual?

3. Have you or someone you care for:

a. Lost interest in friends, hobbies, or other activities that were once enjoyable?

b. Been resisting change or new activities?

c. Become more upset or angrier than usual?

d. Often felt sad?

Steps toward diagnosis

People with memory loss or other possible warning signs of Alzheimer's may fail to recognize that they have a problem and might resist following up on their symptoms. Signs of dementia may be more obvious to friends and family.

The first step is to find a doctor you feel comfortable with. Your local Alzheimer's Association can assist you with finding a doctor. There is no one type of doctor that specializes in diagnosing and treating this disease. Many people usually contact their primary care doctor about their concerns. Primary care doctors often oversee the diagnostic process themselves.

Another problem people face when diagnosed with this disease is how the doctor or medical profession explains the illness and how the person is told. It's heartbreaking enough for anyone to be told that this is happening to them and that their future is no longer in their control. The Alzheimer's Association suggested this to ease the way for the person and family to understand what is going to happen and to give the person a dignified diagnosis.

1. **Speak to the patient directly—that is the person with dementia.** That is the person with the disease and that is the person who needs to know and understand first.

2. **Tell the truth.** Doctors do not always have all of the answers, but they should be honest about what they do know and why they believe the knowledge they have is the truth.

3. **Test early.** The patient needs an accurate diagnosis as fast as possible, which gives them more time to deal and live to their fullest potential. It gives the person time to get more information about the appropriate clinical trials.

4. **Take the patient's concerns seriously, regardless of their age.** Age may be the biggest risk factor for this disease. It is definitely not a normal part of aging. Do not make the patient feel that their concerns are unfounded or they are old so they do not under-

stand what is happening to them. This disease can hit people in their 40s, 50s, and 60s.

5. **Deliver the news in plain but sensitive language.** This is probably one of the most vital and important things that the patient needs to hear. Using language that the person can understand and being sensitive will help the person feel better and feel that the health care provider is showing compassion for his/her feelings

6. **Coordinate with other care providers.** If the patient is seeing more than one specialist, it is important that the doctors coordinate their information so that any changes in the patient can be identified early on and that they do not have to retake or repeat any tests unnecessarily.

7. **Explain the purpose of different tests and what you hope to learn from them.** These tests can be both physically and emotionally draining. It helps the patient to understand the purpose of all of the tests and the duration of each test, and what you hope to learn from them. There should be an option for the patient to take a breather or a break between tests that are longer in order to ask questions.

8. **What tools are there that you can give the patient in order to cope and live with this disease?** Do not give the patient this diagnosis and leave them alone to deal with it. The person needs to understand what is going to happen to them, and they need to know if there are any medical options and what support services are available for them and their family members.

9. **Work with the patient on a plan for healthy living.** Medication may help modify some of the neurological symptoms. Patients are interested in other recommendations for keeping healthy, like diet, exercise, and social engagements.

10. **Recognize that the patient is an individual and will experience the disease in his/her own or unique way.** This disease affects

each person in different ways and at a different rate. Telling the patient the rate that this illness will affect him/her and how fast things will go downhill needs to be addressed to that patient and not to others in general.

11. **Alzheimer's is a journey, not a destination.** There is no prescription to cure this illness, and doctors need to be their patient's advocate and work with them to get quality care and try to have some type of life while going through these changes.

Stages of Alzheimer's disease

Experts have documented common patterns of symptom progression that occur in many individuals with Alzheimer's disease, and developed several methods of "staging" based on these patterns. Progression of symptoms corresponds in a general way to the underlying nerve cell degeneration that takes place in Alzheimer's disease.

Nerve cell damage typically begins with cells involved in learning and memory and gradually spreads to cells that control other aspects of thinking, judgment, and behavior. The damage eventually affects cells that control and coordinate movement.

Staging systems provide useful frames of reference for understanding how the disease may unfold and for making future plans. But it is important to note that all stages are artificial benchmarks in a continuous process that can vary greatly from one person to another. Not everyone will experience every symptom, and symptoms may occur at different times in different individuals. People with Alzheimer's die an average of four to six years after diagnosis, but the duration of the disease can vary from three to twenty years.

The framework for this fact sheet is a system that outlines key symptoms characterizing seven stages, ranging from unimpaired function to very severe cognitive decline. This framework is based on a system developed by Barry Reisberg, M.D., Clinical Director of the New York University School of Medicine's Silberstein Aging and Dementia Research Center.

Within this framework, we have noted which stages correspond to the widely used concepts of mild, moderate, moderately severe, and severe Alzheimer's disease. We have also noted which stages fall within the more general divisions of early-stage, mid-stage, and late-stage categories.

STAGE 1: NO COGNITIVE IMPAIRMENT

Unimpaired individuals experience no memory problems and none are evident to a health care professional during a medical interview.

STAGE 2: VERY MILD DECLINE

Individuals at this stage feel as if they have memory lapses, forgetting familiar words or names or the location of keys, eyeglasses, or other everyday objects. But these problems are not evident during a medical examination or apparent to friends, family, or co-workers.

STAGE 3: MILD COGNITIVE DECLINE

Early-stage Alzheimer's can be diagnosed in some, but not all, individuals with these symptoms. Friends, family, or co-workers begin to notice deficiencies. Problems with memory or concentration may be measurable in clinical testing or discernible during a detailed medical interview. Common difficulties include:

- Word-or name-finding problems noticeable to family or close associates

- Decreased ability to remember names when introduced to new people

- Performance issues in social and work settings noticeable to others

- Reading a passage and retaining little material

- Losing or misplacing a valuable object

- Decline in ability to plan or organize

STAGE 4: MODERATE COGNITIVE DECLINE

(Mild or early-stage Alzheimer's disease)

At this stage, a careful medical interview detects clear-cut deficiencies in the following areas:

- Decreased knowledge of recent events

- Impaired ability to perform challenging mental arithmetic. For example, to count backward from 100 by 7s

- Decreased capacity to perform complex tasks, such as marketing, planning dinner for guests, or paying bills and managing finances

- Reduced memory of personal history

- The affected individual may seem subdued and withdrawn, especially in socially or mentally challenging situations

STAGE 5: MODERATELY SEVERE COGNITIVE DECLINE
(Moderate or mid-stage Alzheimer's disease)

Major gaps in memory and deficits in cognitive function emerge. Some assistance with day-to-day activities becomes essential. At this stage, individuals may:

- Be unable during a medical interview to recall such important details as their current address, their telephone number, or the name of the college or high school from which they graduated

- Become confused about where they are or about the date, day of the week, or season

- Have trouble with less challenging mental arithmetic; for example, counting backward from 40 by 4s, or from 20 by 2s

- Need help choosing proper clothing for the season or the occasion

- Usually retain substantial knowledge about themselves and know their own name and the names of their spouse or children

- Usually require no assistance with eating or using the toilet

STAGE 6: SEVERE COGNITIVE DECLINE
(Moderately severe or mid-stage Alzheimer's disease)

Memory difficulties continue to worsen, significant personality changes may emerge, and affected individuals need extensive help with daily activities. At this stage, individuals may:

- Lose most awareness of recent experiences and events as well as of their surroundings

- Recollect their personal history imperfectly, although they generally recall their own name

- Occasionally forgets the name of their spouse or primary caregiver, but generally can distinguish familiar from unfamiliar faces

- Need help getting dressed properly; without supervision, may make such errors as putting pajamas over daytime clothes or shoes on wrong feet

- Experience disruption of their normal sleep/waking cycle

- Need help with handling details of toileting (flushing toilet, wiping and disposing of tissue properly)

- Have increasing episodes of urinary or fecal incontinence

- Experience significant personality changes and behavioral symptoms, including suspiciousness and delusions (for example, believing that their caregiver is an impostor); hallucinations (seeing or hearing things that are not really there); or compulsive, repetitive behaviors such as hand-wringing or tissue shredding

- Tend to wander and become lost

STAGE 7: VERY SEVERE COGNITIVE DECLINE
(Severe or late-stage Alzheimer's disease)

This is the final stage of the disease when individuals lose the ability to respond to their environment, the ability to speak, and, ultimately, the ability to control movement.

- Frequently individuals lose their capacity for recognizable speech, although words or phrases may occasionally be uttered

- Individuals need help with eating and toileting, and there is general incontinence

- Individuals lose the ability to walk without assistance, then the ability to sit without support, the ability to smile, and the ability to hold their head up. Reflexes become abnormal and muscles grow rigid. Swallowing is impaired.

Telling Others About An Alzheimer Diagnosis

When you learn that someone you care about has Alzheimer's, you may hesitate to tell the person that he or she has the disease. You may also have a hard time deciding whether to tell family and friends. Once you are emotionally ready to discuss the diagnosis, how will you break the news? Here are some suggestions for talking about the disease with others.

RESPECT THE PERSON'S RIGHT TO KNOW

- You may want to protect the person by withholding information. But your loved one is an adult with the right to know the truth. It can be a relief to hear the diagnosis, especially if the person had suspected he or she has Alzheimer's disease.

- In many cases, people who are diagnosed early are able to participate in important decisions about their healthcare and legal and financial planning.

- While there is no current cure for Alzheimer's, life will not stop with the diagnosis. There are treatments and services that can make life better for everyone.

PLAN HOW TO TELL THE PERSON

- Talk with doctors, social workers and others who work with people who have Alzheimer's to plan an approach for discussing the diagnosis.

- Consider a "family conference" to tell the person about the diagnosis. He or she may not remember the discussion, but may remember that people cared enough to come together. You may need to have more than one meeting to cover the details.

- Shape the discussion to fit the person's emotional state, medical condition, and ability to remember and make decisions.

- Pick the best time to talk about the diagnosis. People with Alzheimer's may be more receptive to new information at different times of the day.

- Don't provide too much information at once. Listen carefully to the person. They often signal the amount of information they can deal with through their questions and reactions. Later, you can explain the symptoms of Alzheimer's and talk about planning for the future and getting support.

HELP THE PERSON ACCEPT THE DIAGNOSIS

- The person may not understand the meaning of the diagnosis or may deny it. Accept such reactions and avoid further explanations.

- If they respond well, try providing additional information.

- The person with Alzheimer's may forget the initial discussion but not the emotion involved. If telling them upsets them, hearing additional details may trigger the same reaction later.

- Reassure your loved one. Express your commitment to help and give support. Let the person know that you will do all you can to keep your lives fulfilling.

- Be open to the person's need to talk about the diagnosis and his or her emotions.

- Look for nonverbal signs of sadness, anger or anxiety. Respond with love and reassurance.

- Encourage the person to join a support group for individuals with memory loss. Your local Alzheimer's Association can help you locate a group. To find an Association near you, please call 1.800.272.3900 or go to www.alz.org.

TELLING FAMILY AND FRIENDS

An Alzheimer diagnosis doesn't only affect the person receiving it. The lives of family members and friends may also drastically change.

- Be honest with family and friends about the person's diagnosis. Explain that Alzheimer's is a brain disease, not a psychological or emotional disorder.

- Share educational materials from the Alzheimer's Association. The more that people learn about the disease, the more comfortable they may feel around the person.

- Invite family to support groups sponsored by your local Alzheimer's Association.

- Realize that some people may drift out of your life, as they may feel uncomfortable around the person or may not want to help provide care.

- Alzheimer's disease can also impact children and teens. Just as with any family member, be honest about the person's diagnosis with the young people in your life. Encourage them to ask questions.

Publications and Organizations

NINDS Dementia Information Page. Dementia information page compiled by the National Institute of Neurological Disorders and Stroke (NINDS).

Dementia: Hope Through Research. Information booklet about Alzheimer's disease, vascular dementia, and other types of dementia compiled by the National Institute of Neurological Disorders and Stroke (NINDS).

NINDS Multi-Infarct Dementia Information Page. Multi-infarct dementia information sheet compiled by the National Institute of Neurological Disorders and Stroke (NINDS).

NINDS Dementia With Lewy Bodies Information Page. Dementia With Lewy Bodies information sheet compiled by the National Institute of Neurological Disorders and Stroke (NINDS).

Myoclonus Fact Sheet. Myoclonus fact sheet compiled by the National Institute of Neurological Disorders and Stroke (NINDS).

Creutzfeldt-Jakob Disease Fact Sheet. Creutzfeldt-Jakob Disease (CJD) fact sheet compiled by the National Institute of Neurological Disorders and Stroke (NINDS).

ALZHEIMER ORGANIZATIONS

Alzheimer's Disease Education and Referral Center (ADEAR)
National Institute on Aging
P.O. Box 8250
Silver Spring, MD 20907-8250
adear@nia.nih.gov
www.nia.nih.gov/alzheimers
Tel: 1-800-438-4380
Fax: 301-495-3334

National Institute of Mental Health
National Institutes of Health, DHHS
6001 Executive Blvd. Rm. 8184, MSC 9663
Bethesda, MD 20892-9663
nimhinfo@nih.gov
www.nimh.nih.gov
Tel: 301-443-4513/866-415-8051
301-443-8431 (TTY)

Alzheimer's Association
225 North Michigan Avenue, Floor 17
Chicago, IL 60601-7633
info@alz.org
www.alz.org
Tel: 312-335-8700
1-800-272-3900 (24-hour helpline)
TDD: 312-335-5886

Alzheimer's Foundation of America
322 Eighth Avenue
7th Floor
New York, NY 10001
info@alzfdn.org
www.alzfdn.org
Tel: 866-AFA-8484 (232-8484)

National Organization for Rare Disorders (NORD)
55 Kenosia Avenue
Danbury, CT 06810
orphan@rarediseases.org
www.rarediseases.org
Tel: 203-744-0100
Voice Mail 800-999-NORD (6673)

Family Caregiver Alliance/ National Center on Caregiving
785 Market St., Suite 750
San Francisco, CA 94103
info@caregiver.org
www.caregiver.org
Tel: 415-434-3388 800-445-8106

Association for Frontotemporal Degeneration (AFTD)
Radnor Station Building #2 Suite 320
290 King of Prussia Road
Radnor, PA 19087
info@theaftd.org
www.theaftd.org
Tel: 267-514-7221 866-507-7222

National Family Caregivers Assn.
10400 Connecticut Avenue, Suite 500
Kensington, MD 20895-3944
info@thefamilycaregiver.org
www.thefamilycaregiver.org
Tel: 800-896-3650

Well Spouse Association
63 West Main Street, Suite H
Freehold, NJ   07728
info@wellspouse.org
www.wellspouse.org
Tel: 800-838-0879 732-577-8899

National Respite Network and Resource Center
800 Eastowne Drive, Suite 105
Chapel Hill, NC 27514
http://www.archrespite.org
Tel: 919-490-5577 x222

BrightFocus Foundation
22512 Gateway Center Drive
Clarksburg, MD   20871
info@brightfocus.org
www.brightfocus.org/alzheimers/
Tel: 1- 800-437-2423

National Hospice and Palliative Care Organization /National Hospice Foundation
1731 King Street
Alexandria, VA   22314
nhpco_info@nhpco.org
www.nhpco.org
Tel: 703-837-1500 Helpline: 800-658-8898

Alzheimer's Drug Discovery Foundation
57 West 57th Street, Suite 904
New York, NY   10019
info@alzdiscovery.org
www.alzdiscovery.org
Tel: 212-901-8000

John Douglas French Alzheimer's Foundation
11620 Wilshire Blvd., Suite 270
Los Angeles, CA   90025
www.jdfaf.org
Tel: 310-445-4650

Lewy Body Dementia Association
912 Killian Hill Road, S.W.
Lilburn, GA   30047
lbda@lbda.org
www.lbda.org
Tel: Telephone: 404-935-6444 LBD
Caregiver Link: 800-539-9767

National Institute on Aging
Building 31, Room 5C27
31 Center Drive, MSC 2292
Bethesda, MD 20892
www.nia.nih.gov/alzheimers/topics/caregiving
Tel: 1-800-222-2225

PART FOUR

Family Memories

CHAPTER 14

Because We Love You Mom, Here Are Our Words

In this part of the book, I have asked many of my family members and my mother's friends to write what they remember about the good times they had with her before she got sick.

————

In Dad's words: Wherever you are, dear Ruth, whenever I pen a special rhyme, remember I will always love you: TILL THE END OF TIME!

————

I read this to my mom on her last Mother's Day.

Dear Mom:

Reading has always been the way for me to escape to other worlds, learn about many different places, and expand my knowledge of so many subjects. With a note pad in hand and several pens at the ready, I begin reading the many books that authors send me each day. Detailing the plot, the characters, and taking notes throughout, I create a perfect analysis of the book before beginning my review. Remembering what you told me, to always look for that special message in the book and create that first paragraph to stimulate reader interest, I begin my review.

Perfection: that's what you always told me. Each piece of writing, each assignment had to be done to the standards set by my teachers and professors, and then pass the highest test: Yours. I even remember coming out of school one night and you stuck your hand out, waiting to see what I got on my midterm in one of my graduate courses in administration. I still smile when I remember what happened. I left out one question and got a ninety-eight, and I told you what I did wrong and the right answer. But, the professor was so frustrated with most of the other students that she had to revamp the scores by adding ten points to everyone's test scores just to have more students pass. So, you were satisfied with my 108, and of course on the final I did get 100 and an A in the class, because it was what was expected of me by myself, and of course you.

Till this day I still create my reviews, my schedule for my radio show, and anything else that I decide to venture into—like the *MJ Magazine* in memory of Marcia Joyce— with the understanding that my work has to stand up to the highest standards, and the articles, reviews, stories, and issues that are published should be equal to those of any credible magazine on the newsstands.

So, Mom, it's three years today and it seems like yesterday. I hope it will continue to make you proud of me. You taught me well. Yes, I never leave the house without looking my best. You were my mom, my mentor, and my best friend. You will always be here for me in spirit.

Love, Frani and Keith

Before my sister passed away she wrote this special poem:

A Very Special Poem

by Marcia Wallach, daughter of Ruth Swerdloff

Around the corner I have a friend,
in this great city that has no end.
Yet the days go by and weeks rush on,
and before I know it, a year is gone.

I never see my old friend's face,
for life is a swift and terrible race.
She knows I like her just as well,
and in the days when I rang her bell,
And she rang mine; but we were younger then,
and now we are busy tired women.

Tired of playing a foolish game,
tired of trying to make a name.
"Tomorrow" I say! I will call on her,
just to show that I'm thinking of her and she is not a blur.
But tomorrow comes and tomorrow goes,
and distance between us grows and grows.

Around the corner, yet miles away.
Here's a telegram miss, "Your friend died today."
And that's what we get and deserve in the end,
a very dear and vanished friend.

Remember to always say what you mean. If you love someone, tell him or her. Don't be afraid to express yourself; reach out and tell someone what he or she means to you, because when you decide that it is the right time, it might be too late. Seize the day.

Never have regrets. And most importantly, stay close to your friends and family, for they have helped make you the person you are today.

Doing It Her Way — My Mom, Ruth Swerdloff

My mom was the taxi driver of our family. She was the person my sister and I would call if we needed a ride to anywhere. Although our friends' moms were great, our mom was the one who always said yes. She would do pickups late at night, and deliveries early in the morning. Nothing was ever too hard for her. I remember quite a few times, when my brother was staying at my home, he would decide that it was time to go home and my mom would drive out to Long Island at 11:00 P.M. to pick him up. Like I said, nothing was ever too hard for her for any of her children.

Mom would be the one to sit and listen for hours when anyone had a problem. She was the mom everyone came to, the mom with understanding, the mom with patience. It was great growing up and having her as a mom.

I remember one day, as an adult, Mom and I decided to spend the day together. I had driven into the Bronx, where Mom lives, and we went out for lunch. She then decided that she would like to take a ride up to see my brother where he worked. We would only stop by for a minute. She insisted that she drive.

As we came upon the intersection, there was a big sign that said No Left Turns. My mom insisted that it was okay because she had done it before. I reminded her that it was a new sign, and that she shouldn't make the turn. Mom, being mom, doing it her way, insisted that it was okay.

We pulled into the parking lot of where my brother worked, and who pulled in right behind us? A police officer. Sitting in the car with him was a very large German shepherd. The police officer got out of his car, came over to Mom, and said "Lady, you're not allowed to make that turn—license and registration, please, I'm giving you a ticket." Mom being mom literally pulled out three different wallets looking for her license. She looked at him with the sweetest smile, and said, "I know it's here someplace–just give me a few seconds." A few seconds turned into a few minutes, a few minutes turned into twenty minutes. She went through wallet one, then two, and by the time she pulled out wallet three, the police officer was getting quite impatient. He just looked at her and said, "Lady, let this be a warning to you. Please don't do it again." He and his big dog left and Mom never did get the ticket. We laughed about it the rest of the day. It was a sight to see, having Mom pull out all these wallets while the police officer just stood there waiting. I guess you would have had to be there.

I miss the way Mom and I would spend the day together, laughing, talking, and joking. However, in one respect I'm lucky; I have wonderful memories of my mom the way she used to be before dementia took over. I wonder what she remembers, if anything. Hopefully, somewhere in her mind, she too remembers the wonderful times we all had together.

With much love always,
Your daughter, Marcia

A Night To Remember

By Jamie Miller, Ruth's Granddaughter

I was asked to write something special about my grandmother. One thing I said…how can I just narrow it down to one thing? My aunt said to write about a special moment that you could remember the most. One memory stands out in my mind every time I think of this amazing woman.

When I was seven years old, we used to go up to the country every summer to a place called Breezy Corners. This summer was very different; this was the summer of the accident! My brother Jason, a bunch of kids, and I were playing in the back of our bungalow, and one of the kids had a toy water rocket. The rocket was supposed to shoot up in the air, and instead shot into my eye. I was crying my eyes out and my five-year-old brother ran home. Before I knew it, everyone I had known was standing there.

A doctor, who of course said I needed a hospital, my mother, and grandmother were freaking out. Well, the best hospitals were hours away, but my grandmother drove for hours until she found the best hospital for my needs. She was stopping and calling every hospital on the way. We finally found a hospital in the city, and when we got there my grandmother held me all night long. I remember until this day lying on her shoulder. I couldn't see out of my eye at all, but I remember her shoulder and her stroking my hair, telling me everything was going to be okay.

I needed a lot of surgeries and doctor appointments following the accident. To make sure I went to every appointment, she bribed me with baby dolls. My grandmother came to every single one. She sat at the hospital every day, even though I couldn't see her. My mother and grandmother would tell me what was on TV because I had patches on my eyes.

My grandmother is and always will be an amazing grandmother. She might not remember me with her words and her mind, but when she looks at me, her eyes tell me otherwise. Words cannot describe just how much I love my grandmother now, forever, and always.

Who Is Next?

by Fran Lewis

The lives of so many people have been turned inside out.
The lives of so many people have changed for the worse, no doubt.
Their lives were normal just like yours and mine.
Their lives were normal one minute and the next far from fine.

It sneaks up slowly without a single clue.
It sneaks up slowly inside anyone, even you.
Without a hint or even a word you begin to forget and then,
You start to act as if you don't know what, where, or when.

You forget your keys, your phone number and more.
You have no idea that the worst is still in store.
You're driving a car and you forget which way
You travel to work each and every day.

Pulling over to the side you begin to cry
Because you can't remember the way, even if you try
Starting to write lists each morning to help you know
What the day has in store for you while on the go.

And just when you think it could not get any worse,
You go shopping at the market and forget where you left your purse.
You look around and try to think of where it might be,
Not even realizing as you look that it's on your arm where it should be.

What could be causing your memory to go?
Dementia of course is about to make you slow
Down in your actions, your thoughts, and your life.
It enjoys creeping into your mind to bring you strife.

It slowly eats away at you each day
Making your life difficult in most every way.
Eating before leaving and going to the store,
You stop for pizza and a whole lot more.

You don't remember that you just had tea.
You don't remember that you ate with me.
Then you forget the names of so many who are dear.
That's scares you into going to the doctor to learn your worst fear.

Yes, it's the start of that dreaded disease.
It will overtake you in time and with ease.
The doctor tells you that you have the start of this disease.
Yes, Alzheimer's has started to pick at your brain with much ease.

Sorry to tell you there is little we can do
To stop this disease from destroying you.
I sat in the doctor's office and cried.
I sat in his office and tried and tried

Not to react when he said these words to my mom,
Watching her not understand how come.
By the time they realized it was too late.
By the time they realized she could not tell you the date.

Not even the city and state where she lives or her address.
It slowly eats away at your dignity to turn your life into a mess
Stem cell research is going on all over the world we know.
The type of research that might make it disappear and just go.

In time maybe there will be an FDA approved drug or cure,
Before it is too late and grief too many will still have to endure.
From me to you and anyone else you need to remember this
Having the person at home and caring for them is truly bliss.

My family loves our mom, no doubt, and we make sure she is safe.
Keeping your loved one at home is the best choice I know.

To anyone who has a loved one with this disease, you need to hang tough and remember the good times that you had with this person and tell them that you love them every day. My mom sees me in the morning when I come down to give her the medications and anything else she needs each day. The first thing she says is "I love you. Do you love me too?" Fortunately, she does know who her children are and she even remembers some other family members. As long as she is on this earth and my family and I can see her, we are still truly blessed. We cannot and will not let this disease overtake our spirits and our hearts, even though it is trying hard to destroy so many minds.

She has had this illness for over six years, and most of the time she cannot remember my name or anyone else's. The only name she remembers is her own. She is a remarkable person. I guess it is my sense of humor that I inherited from my dad that helps keep my spirits up and a smile on my face.

Fran Lewis

If you believe in Miracles, please read this special poem:

God was watching over us
The Flight To Remember

by Fran Lewis

When my mom got sick in 1994
I had no idea what would be in store.
She was so ill she had to have open heart
Surgery that would take her whole chest apart.

It all began with the Leer Jet from hell you see,
Two pilots and a paramedic who were miserable to both my mom and me.
The plane took off from Teterboro, in nine inches of snow,
For a five-hour ride to USCD in California to save her life you know.

But, as soon as we took off the pilots looked at a map and tried to stay cool
In reality the plane was being piloted by a dangerous fool
Not really concerned about my mom at all.
The pilots and paramedic were drinking coffee and having a ball.

Not once did they care about whether we were all right.
This I knew would result in a big fight.
When my mom asked for ice chips and for water, you see,
The paramedic over medicated her right in front of me.

This led to words between us and I told him this too,
"You better make sure that you tell me what you give her before you do."
But, before things got worse the pilot did land,
Causing me to fall out of my seat and hurt my hand.

The seats on this plane did not really exist…
I was sitting on something smaller than my wrist.
Not only wasn't there food, water, or a bathroom on this flight…
Imagine the pilot handing you a bedpan and you having to go sitting upright.
With three blankets over my head I tried to not get too wet.
I thought about the indignity and still another chink in the net.
I could not believe what happened after we finally did land;
The door of the plane fell on the pilot and broke his hand.
I did not know whether to laugh or cry.
I just looked at him and felt no pity; I bet you could figure out why.

A gray haired man alighted from another Leer Jet I saw.
He said he was the president of the company. I told him the score.
I asked if his plane was in good operating order to fly.
He asked what the question was for and I told him why.

"You see my mom is quite sick," and I told him the bare facts.
I told him the problems and what his airline lacked.
He went to a phone while I used one of his,
Calling my brother to stop the 12, 500 dollar check for his biz.

They had to get a new pilot to replace the one with the broken hand.
Hopefully they would find one who could go up and safely land.
Well, a trip that was supposed to take six hours or less, but no more
Took sixteen hours, and I was out to settle a score.

We landed in the middle of the night in an airport that you could barely see,
With an ambulance waiting and another paramedic who greeted me.
We went to the hospital and settled my mom with the staff.
I saw the paramedics, who did nothing but laugh.

The next morning I was called to the hospital because she was really bad.
The staff that greeted me looked upset and really scared.
They said they were not sure whether we got there in time.
I refused to believe it and told them I knew she would be fine.

Never before had they met anyone like me, they said,
Looking at me with eyes that only had dread.
The doctors and nurses at UCSD I will never forget
They saved her life and I guess the flight from hell I cannot regret.
She is still here and my family is grateful to them you know.
Unfortunately, Alzheimer's got her six years ago.
Miracles do happen, and I believe that is true.
I hope that there is a cure in my lifetime, and hers too.

Alzheimer's-Free: Imagine That!

Imagine finding a cure for this dreaded illness so that my family and many others will never have to deal with this ever again. What if one doctor somewhere in the world found the key? I can imagine it, and I hope that it is not too far in the future. So, here are my words, and I hope that somehow God will hear them and know that the world is waiting for one more miracle, and we hope that it happens soon.

I pray everyday for a cure for this disease. I wish that just one more time I could have a real conversation with my mom and tell her all of the things that I have accomplished since she became ill. I have no one to share all of my accomplishments with the way I did with her. To anyone who has had to deal with this dreaded disease I wish the same for you. JUST ONE MORE MIRACLE!

Fran Lewis

Just One Miracle

Just one more miracle is all I asked of you.
Just one more time to speak with my mom like I used to do.
One more time to tell her about my day.
One more time to talk to her in our special way.

Just one more miracle to find a cure, you see.
One more miracle, not just for me but also for others who need hope to be
Like they were before…working and living their lives so true,
Hoping that their minds will be restored and a life like me and you.

But, I know that it is a dream that I wished for so long.
It hurts to see my mom and others who are no longer strong.
Someday I hope that the world will hear their voices
When there are medications of which they will have choices.

To restore what has happened to their memories and minds.
To restore who they were with these miracle cure and finds.

That no one will ever have to grieve for a loved one who has been hit
With Alzheimer's disease, which destroys you, bit by bit.

Just one more miracle, I know you can do if for everyone you see.
Just one more miracle, not just for me but also for others who will be

Joyous and grateful if you can do this for all of us.
Joyous and grateful and for you we will truly fuss.
Never taking it for granted if you find a way to show
That Alzheimer's is out and clear minds are what we will only know.
1.

Fran Remembers

My mom has always been a force to be reckoned with. She decided my wardrobe from the day I was born. I remember one morning when I went down to have coffee with her before going to school. She looked at me and said, "You cannot go to school in that outfit. Your skirt is too short and your shoes do not match." I just stared at her and said I had no time to change and I was going to be late.

She picked up the phone and called my school and told them I would be late for my first reading class, which started at 7:30 in the morning, because I had to go upstairs and change into a proper outfit to teach children reading. My principal, who did not know whether to laugh or cry, agreed with her and told me to go up and change. "If your mother disapproves of what you are wearing so will I." Needless to say I did change and had to meet her approval before I could go to work.

Another memory involves me going to kindergarte. One morning my teacher was absent. The assistant principal was taking over the class, and she scared me and the other kids, too. In order to protect myself and the other kids from the mean lady, I made my mom sit in class with me all morning.

Kindergarten was only a half a day, and she was wearing her pajamas under her leather jacket and pants. She didn't know she'd have to sit there all morning. She wasn't happy about it, but my grandmother told her not punish me because if someone scared me she had to pay the price and protect her sweet child. Besides, my grandmother told her she should've gotten properly dressed before walking me to school. Thanks Grandma Kati. She always came to my rescue. Boy, could I use her now!

I also remember when mom took me to dancing school and told me it would help me lose weight. All I wanted to do was read a good book or walk with my friends to synagogue on Saturday, and then have lunch with my grandfather when he came from synagogue, too.

I remember having to try out toe shoes. I needed five people to help me keep my balance and not fall over. I was and still am a total klutz, but mom never gave up on my dancing, even though I did!

When I first started to date she would wait up for me to hear all about the date and whether I'd had a great time. It was just like talking to my best friend, but much better.

This is a memory that my mom told me before she got sick. This is really funny.

When my son Keith was only five months old, my sister-in-law Tommy decided it was time to teach him how to catch a football and a baseball. I was in Florida with my two girls for a much needed rest and she was watching Keith for one week at my apartment. She thought nothing of lying down on the carpet with him and teaching him to throw and catch both a football and a baseball.

Remember, he was only five months old! If I hadn't seen this myself when we came home from vacation, I wouldn't have believed it. She told me this was something that she felt every five month old should know how to do.

You should've seen her face when he actually caught the ball. No wonder he became a great pitcher in Little League Baseball.

I'm still here, hear my voice
Do I know who you are?

I am still here although you have forgotten me.
I am still here. Have you forgotten where I live?
I am still here. I am as lonely as can be.
I am still here with all of the love I have to give.

You were my friends and I did a lot for you.
Whenever you needed my help I was there.
I loved you as family, and you know that is true.
Why is it now that you do not know that I am still here?

I know that I cannot remember your name but I know your face.
I know that I cannot speak clearly but I do have something to say,
Giving my all to everyone no matter what the case.
You have forgotten I exist and am still part of the human race.

My daughters often wonder what has become of some of you.
They see you in the elevator and you turn away from them.
Are you afraid you catch my illness and you will understand it too?
The only way you'll get it is if your family has it in their stem.

I would do so much better if you would come and visit me.
I would be so happy to see you and have coffee and talk.
I would be so happy to try and greet you and we
Could go down to the stores in my chair and while you walk.

But I know that will never happen; I realize that, too
You are too busy and I am nothing to you.
So, be thankful that you are able to cope
With all that life hands out in its wide scope.

I will never be able to do handle things on my own.
I will never be able to speak with you and understand you on the phone.
But, I am still here and I hope you will see
That you need to visit before it is too late for me.

Because We Love You and Care

Dedicated to the memory of my Mum, Enid Ann Porter (1914–2004)

She was my strength and my inspiration through all the years of her life. Despite her suffering she never lost her smile or her love of those around her. She was and always will be, my star!

Nightlight

You never liked the darkness, or the coming of the night,
So I put a lamp upon the wall, to flood the path with light.
And as I took you home each night, the lamp would light the way,
To show you home in safety, at the ending of the day.

In the dreary wintertime, its beacon shone out bright.
Dark afternoons you hated, so the lamp would aid your sight.
Even in the summertime, you loved its welcome glow,
Your private lighthouse guiding you when 'ere you'd come and go.

Though sadly you're no longer here, I feel your presence still,
Whether through the summer heat, or 'midst the winter chill.
I look up to the night sky, and wonder at each star,
If you're up there looking down I wonder where you are.

And if at night you're looking down I wonder if you see
This tiny part of God's own world, I wonder if you see me.
I wonder if you see the glow of the lamp that burns so bright,
For I still switch it on each evening, Mum, just so you can see the light.

More Special Dedications

I have asked friends, relatives, and authors, and anyone who wanted to contribute their thoughts and dedications to anyone who has the illness in their family or has died from Alzheimer's. Let their voices ring out and let us band together and let the world know WE WANT A CURE!

———

Uncle Dave and Aunt Ruth

by Mark And Carol Swerdloff,
Fran's Best Friends And Cousins Growing Up

The memories of my Uncle Dave (Doc, may he rest in loving peace) and my Aunt Ruth (and she should live and be well for 120 years) of being kind, generous, good natured, loving, family oriented, humorous, and caring to family and friends will remain in our minds and thoughts for eternity. God bless them both.

This poem is dedicated to my mom and in memory of my dad, who both Mark and Carol spent many hours of fun and love with at their home in Coney Island when they were growing up. This poem is for everyone who has lost someone to this disease, or misses a loved one who has moved away or is no longer here. Thank you to my special cousins Mark and Carol Swerdloff for this amazing and heartfelt tribute.

You can shed tears that her mind is gone,
Or you can smile because she lives.

You can close your eyes and pray that her mind will come back,
Or you can open your eyes and see all she has given.

Your heart can be empty because you can't see her as she was,
Or your heart can be full of the love you have shared.

You can turn your back on tomorrow and live yesterday,
Or you can be happy for tomorrow because of yesterday and today.
You can remember that her mind is gone,
Or you can cherish her memories and let them live on.

You can cry and close your mind,
Be empty and turn your back....
Or you can do what she would want you to do,
Smile, open your eyes, love, and go on.

―――

Aunt Ruth

My Aunt Ruth was an amazing woman. She was always helping others, driving others. The list is too long to mention everything. The best is that my Aunt Ruth was a second mother to me. My mom worked as a teacher and I always had a place to go until my mom came home.

There is something I remember. When my daughter, Faith, got hurt she drove us to the hospital and held her while she received stitches on her head.

I loved my Aunt Ruth and was so lucky to have her in my life.

— Susan Ross

―――

Sharing Stella

by Shari Saia

Have you ever found yourself wondering where you left your eyeglasses or your car keys? You find you know the person you want to introduce to a friend, but suddenly cannot think of his/her name? We all forget things, it's normal. Even as children we were forgetful, leaving our lunch or homework at home or on the bus was not uncommon.

As we age, we become more forgetful. The forgetfulness described I just described is a nuisance, but it's not a serious condition. If the forgetfulness progresses, though, it could be something serious like Alzheimer's disease. My sister-in-law Stella has just been diagnosed with this horrible disease.

I must share Stella with you. My husband is the tenth child of a family of fifteen. Stella is the third eldest. Stella and I have always been close, possibly because she lives so close to my son, Garth, whom I visit as often as I can.

I invited Stella and her caretaker, her unmarried daughter Francis, to come for a weekend at my home. Stella came in the doorway, did not recognize us, and had to be introduced to her brother—my husband—and me. She walked over to me, hugged me, called me "Beautiful," and referred to me with that name throughout the entire weekend, even though I reiterated my name.

Other family members came to visit and she again needed to be introduced to people she had known all of her life. Stella began to "flirt" with my husband, Phil, and Francis said to her, "Phil is your brother." It would've been a comic moment except that Stella grabbed my hands, and for one lucid moment looked into my eyes and pleading said, "Why can't I remember?"

I had instant tears in my eyes. I felt her moment of fear. As quickly as the moment had come, however, it was gone! I wanted to shout out loud, "Stella! Come On!" (As Marlon Brando did, in the movie, *A Streetcare Named Desire*.)

I sat down with Francis and made some suggestions, both for her mom and for herself, as the caretaker. I suggested that she made a simple album with individual photos of her mom's brothers and sisters, and label them with the name and relationship. I told her she should show this to her mom in the morning and evening, and especially before a visit from one of the family members.

I also suggested that she place a black rug in the doorway at night, to prevent Stella from wandering out the door and getting lost. The sight of the rug might stop her from leaving because she'll think it's a large hole in the floor. (It works!)

The final suggestion I gave her was to check into day care facilities that Stella could attend daily. This would give Stella social time, and allow Francis a little freedom to pursue some personal interests.

Shari Saia MS/CCC-SLP
Lake Worth Middle School

Grandma: You Are So Special
By Dani Nicole Miller

My name is Dani; I am in the third grade and the grandchild of Great Grandma Ruth…the best great grandmother in the world. I don't get to see her that often due to the fact that she lives so far away from me, but when I do I love spending time with her.

I feel very close to her. She is my mother's grandmother and I'm named after her husband, David, so I feel a special bond with her. I look at her and I feel love and warmth, and all the things that family means. She can look in my eyes and see just how much I love her.

Sometimes I think she looks at me and sees my mom, and you know what…that's ok too. We all wish that she was 100%, but we are just so happy that she is just still here with us. That way we can still tell her every day, every time we talk to her how much we love her.

I love my Great Grandma Ruth for all the love she gave me and still gives my mother, and all the love she's given to my sister and I.

Thank you Grandma, we love you…XOXOXOXO

———

Special Name, Special Woman

Kati Rose is what they named me, after a very special woman, I hear. My Great Grandmother Ruth had an amazing mommy, so they passed on her name to me, Kati. One amazing woman raising another amazing woman, that's what I hear…I never really got to know my Great Grandmother the stories I heard about her were hilarious and I wish that I had more time with her.

I am going to see her on Friday and I can tell you one thing I am going to hug, kiss, and tell her how much I love her. I love you Grandma Ruth. XOXOXOXO

———

Best Grandma:

by Carly Tappen

I am Carly Megan Tappan and I am eight years old. I love you Grandma Ruth. You are the best grandmother in the whole world. Grandma, I wish I could visit you every day. I live so far away but I think about you all the time. I hope I can see you soon and do stuff with you.

Love ,

Carly, Your great-granddaughter

_____

You're So Special to Me

by Casey Tappen

Great Grandma Ruth, I love you so. Your love and kindness and good heart is what makes you special to me and others. You have been there for me through rain, snow, and even sunny days. We have a special bond and when I think about you my face starts to glow.

When we went to Uncle Keith's and Aunt Marcia's house to see D.J., Josh, and Jake trying to catch fireflies and playing baseball, I remembered how you would play ball with all of us too.

I don't get to see you much because it is such a long distance away and flying in planes is not my favorite thing. But, I would come to see you as much as I could if it would make you happy. It would make my day too. I love you so much and hope to see you soon one day.

Love always,

Your great-granddaughter Casey

Mom: Remember This?

The Day Keith Was Finally Born Mom was Still Making a Fashion Statement

All my life my mom said that we always had to dress our best and look like we were going somewhere. This is a true story about the day my brother Keith was born.

IN RUTH'S OWN WORDS:

I will always remember when I was pregnant with Keith and was going to the hospital to give birth. I did not want to have the baby until I was prepared, properly dressed, and ready. So, I called my brother Kenny and my sister-in-law Tommy to tell them I would not go without the proper nightgowns and sleepwear. The hospital personnel did not know what to think, but I did not care. I was not going to stay there and give birth in their awful hospital gowns.

So, Kenny came with Doc with five nightgowns on hangers, presses, and in plastic bags to the hospital just to make me happy. I did not want to bring Keith into this world with an improperly dressed mother. I also am grateful that he waited to be born on the right day—the same day as his sister Frani. It was really quite thoughtful of him. I told the doctors that any other day would not be acceptable. Of course, Kenny and Doc wanted to leave at that point and pretended not to know me.

But, if anyone knows anything about me, I can do whatever I want and I will always do things my way.

The best medicine, my mom would tell you if she could, is family!
She came alive when her children and grandchildren came to visit. For
anyone who has a family member with Alzheimer's, I hope that this
book helps you gain a better understanding and lets you know you aren't
alone in your struggles.

Fran Lewis

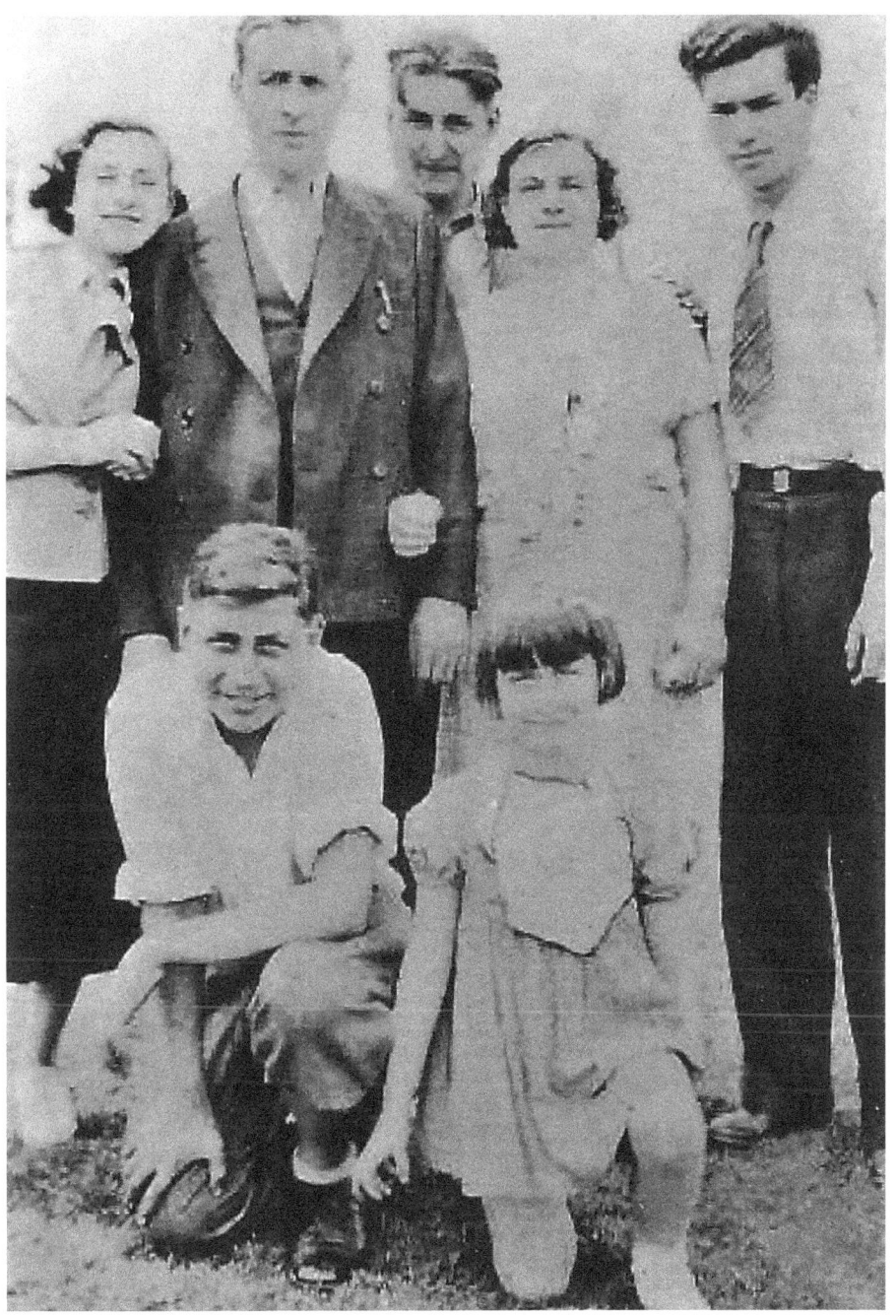

Back row, left to right: Tova, Ruth's sister; Max Goldberg, her father; Harry Goldberg, her brother; Katie Goldberg, her mother; and Irving Goldberg, her brother. Front row: Kenny Goldberg, Ruth's brother and Ruth.

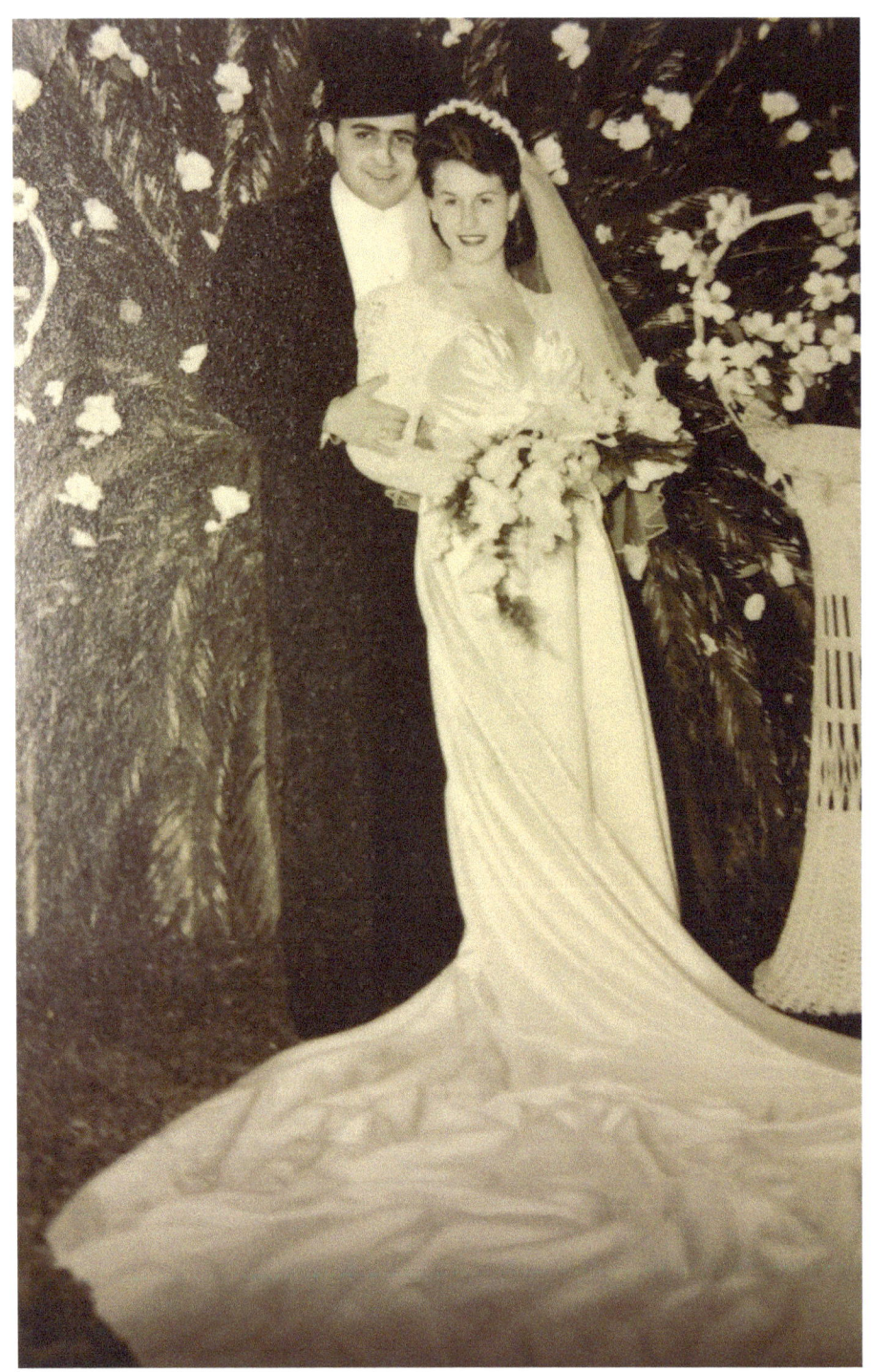

Ruth's wedding picture.

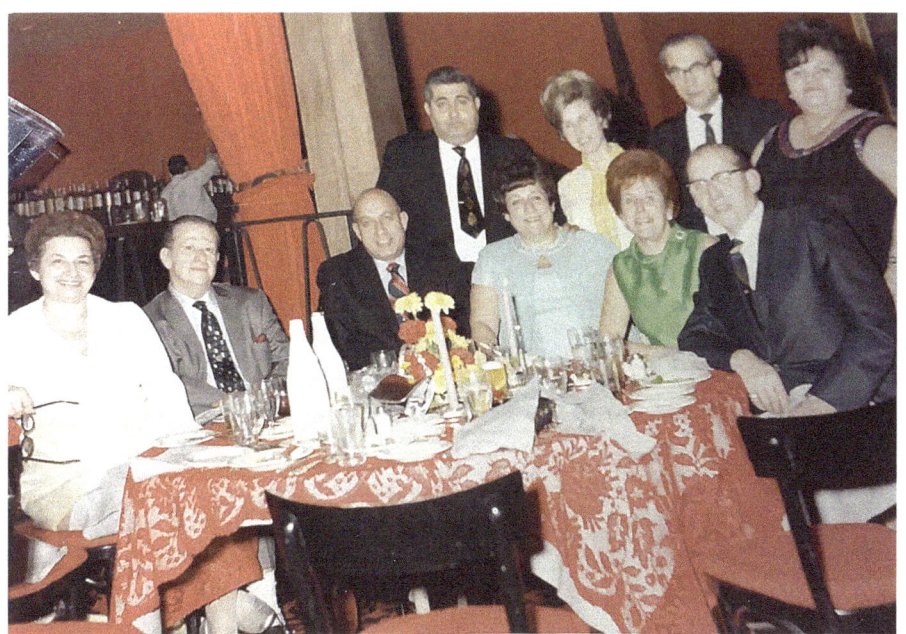

Ruth's sister, brothers and sister-in-laws and her husband.

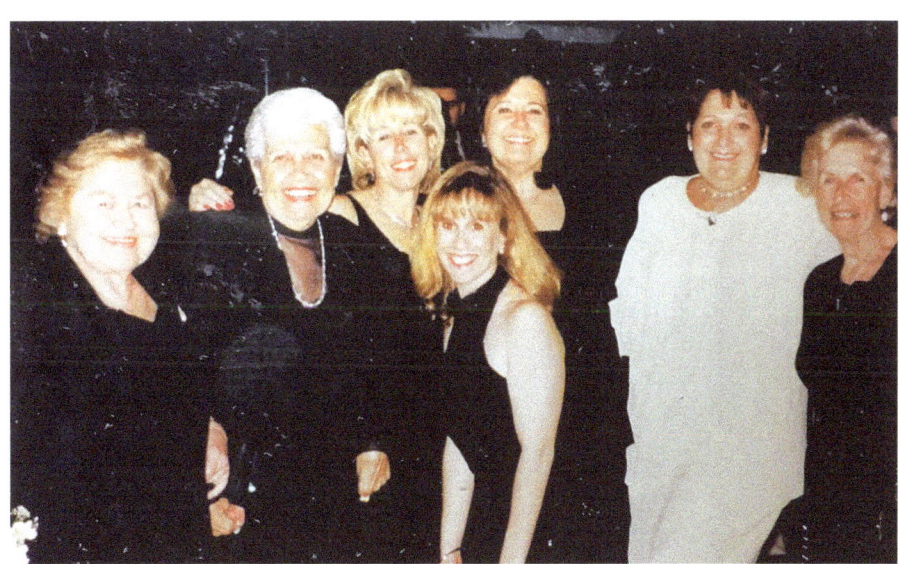

Aunt Judy: sister in law, Aunt Lily: sister in law: Marcia: Daughter in law, Eunice: Niece, and Ruth. Back row: Marcia, Ruth's daughter, and her niece Robin.

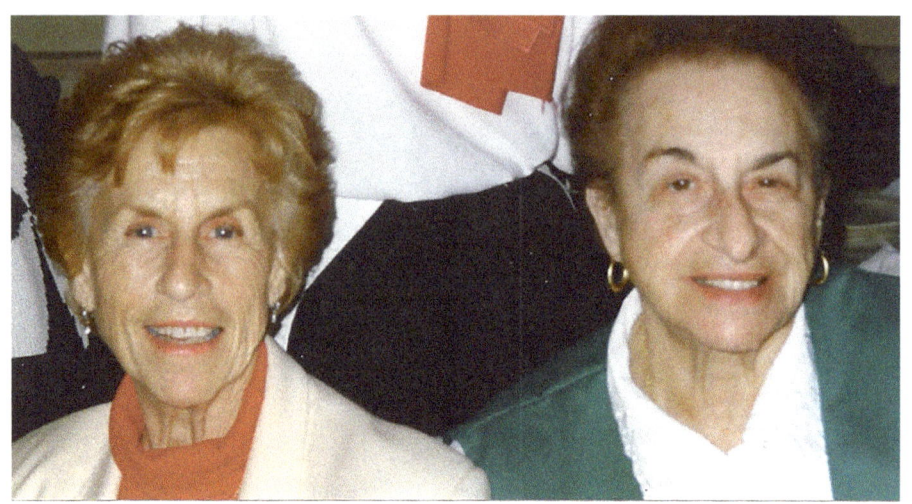

Ruth and her sister Tova.

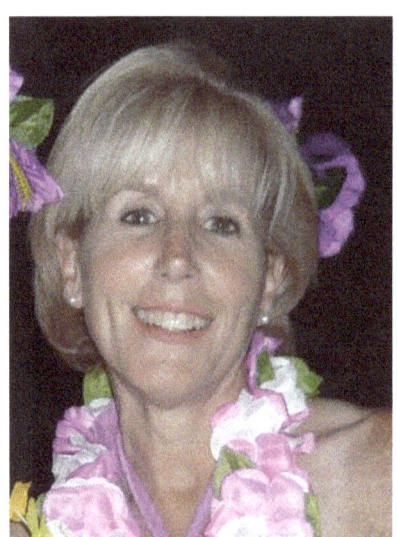

Marcia, Ruth's daughter.

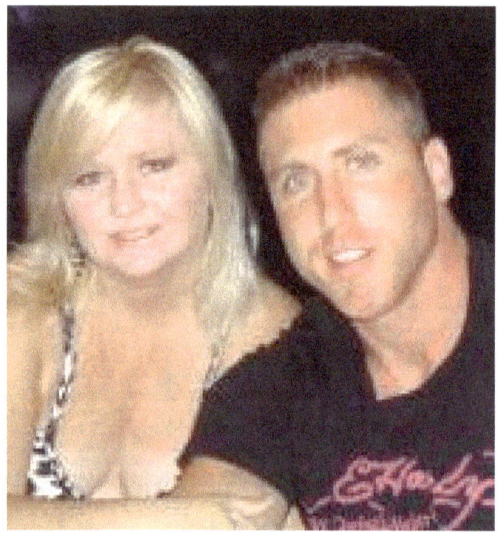

Jason and Tammy, Ruth's grandchildren.

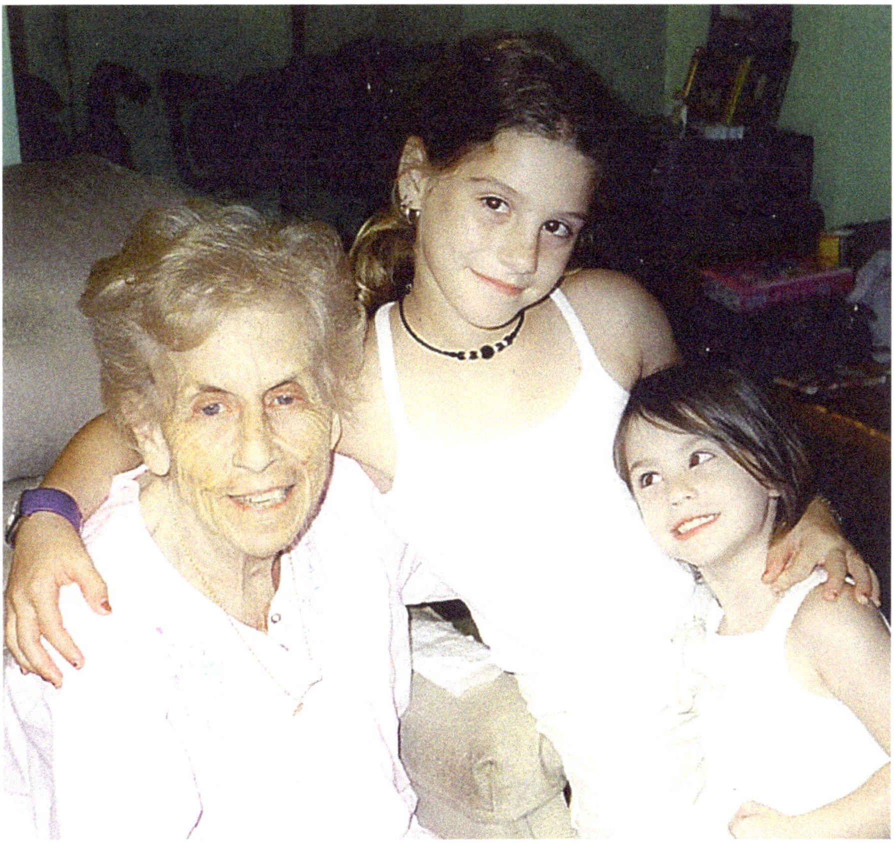

Ruth with Dani Nicole and Kati Rose, her grandchildren.

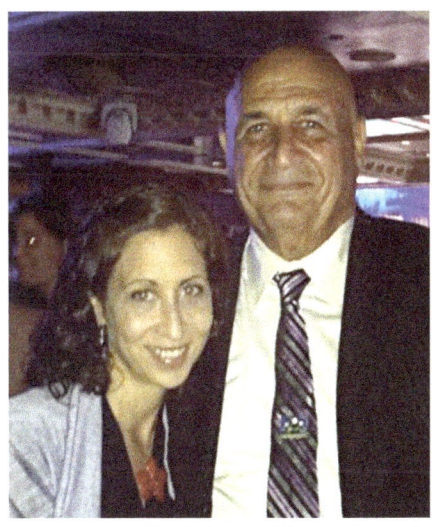

Dayna and Phil, Ruth's niece and nephew.

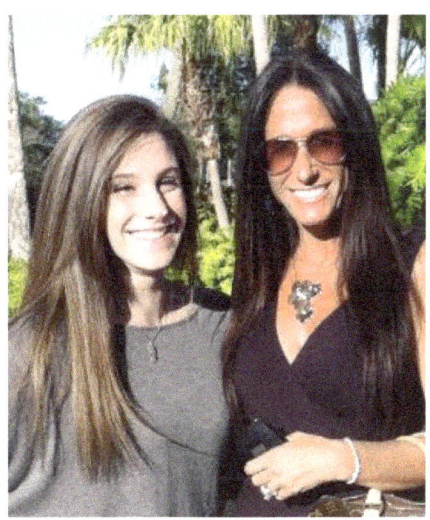

Dani Nicole and Jamie Miller, Ruth's grandchildren.

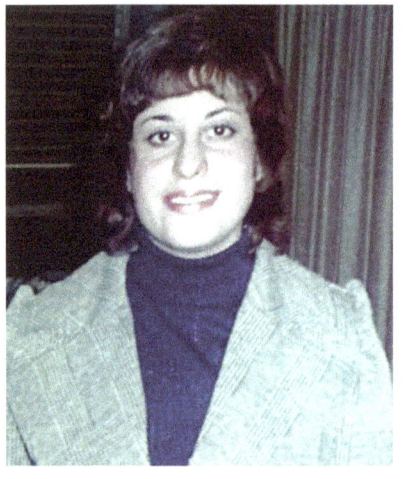

Susan.

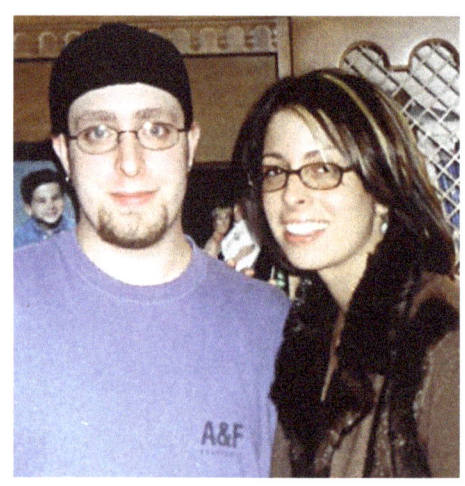

Faith and Jared.

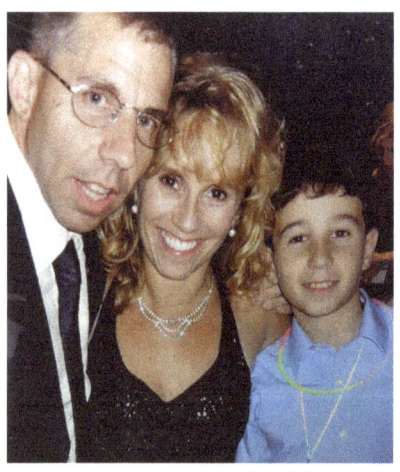

*Her son Keith, with his wife
Marcia and her grandson D.J.*

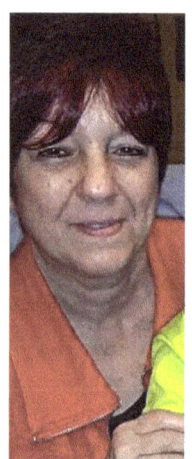

Maria did Ruth's nails.

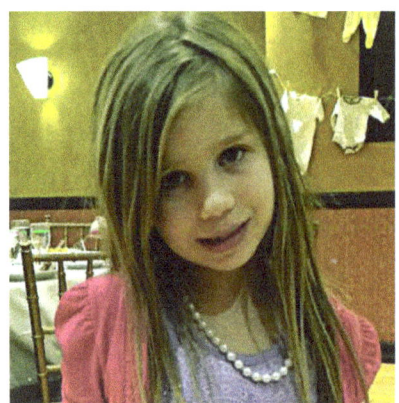

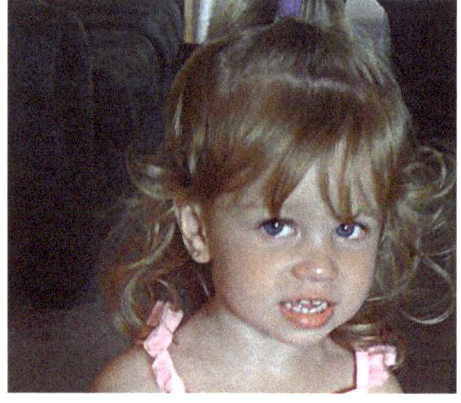

Leah and Olivia, Ruth's great nieces.

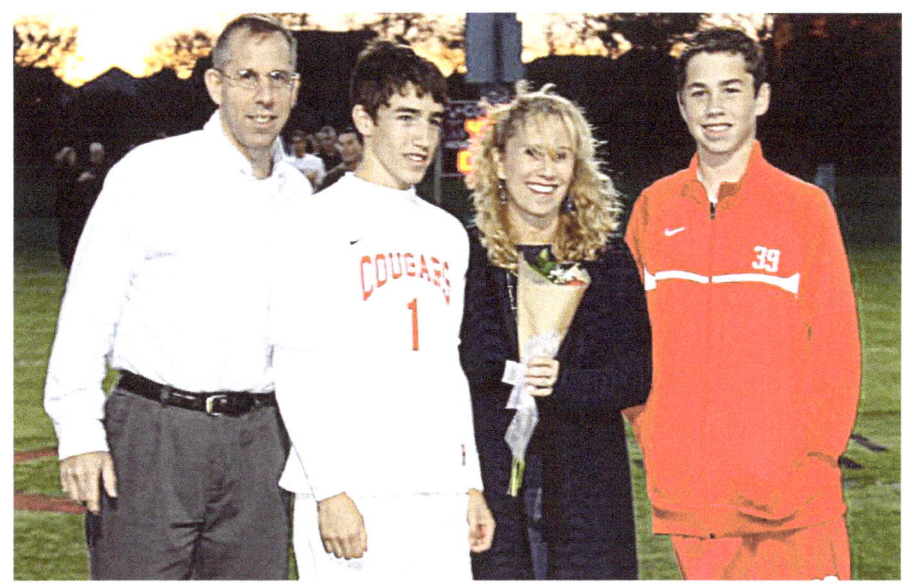

Keith, Ruth's son, and his children Josh and Jake, flanking their mother, Marcia.

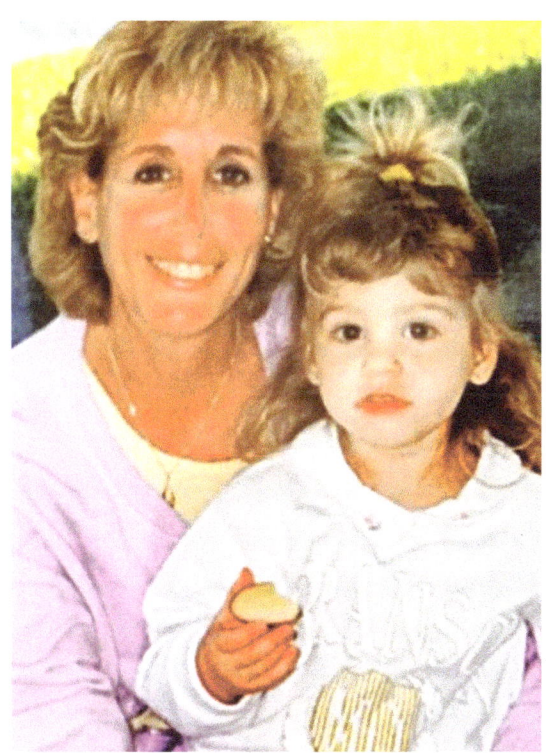

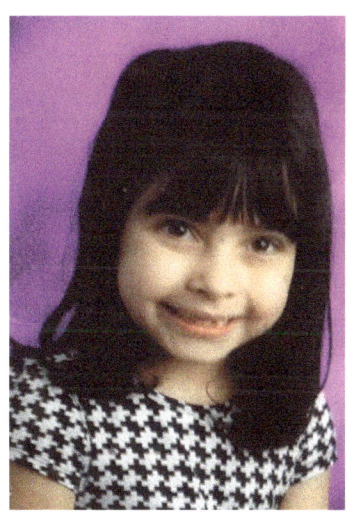

Penelope Mia, Ruth's great niece.

Marcia, Ruth's daughter and Dani, Ruth's granddaughter.

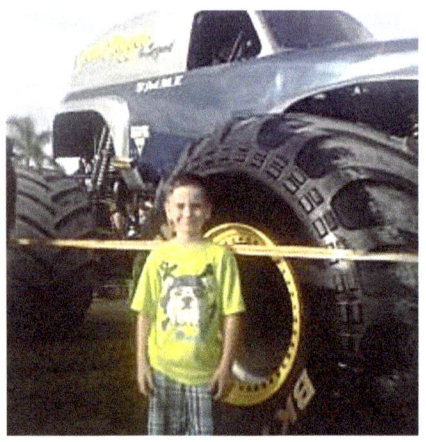

Cade, Ruth's grandson.

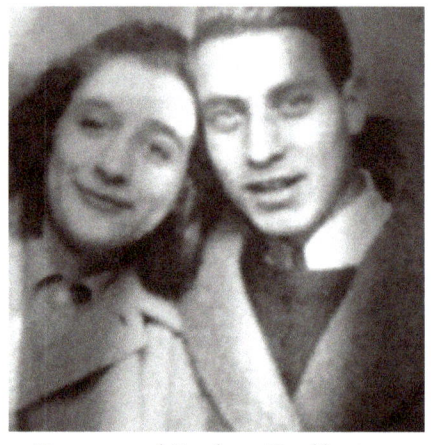

Kenny and Evelyn, Ruth's sister and brother-in-law.

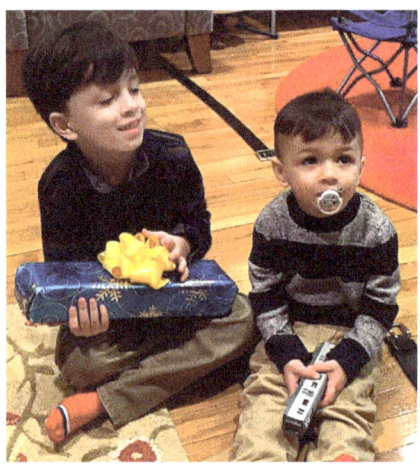

*CW and RT,
Ruth's great-grandchildren*

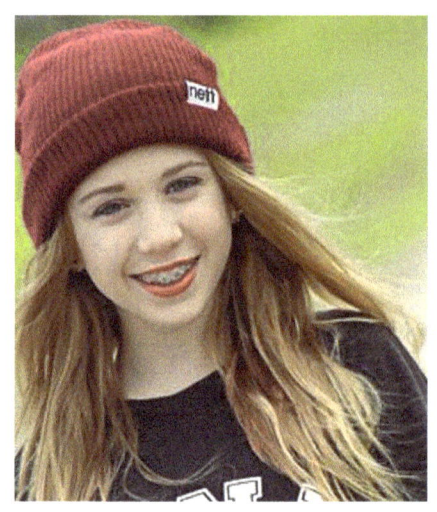

Carly, Ruth's granddaughter.

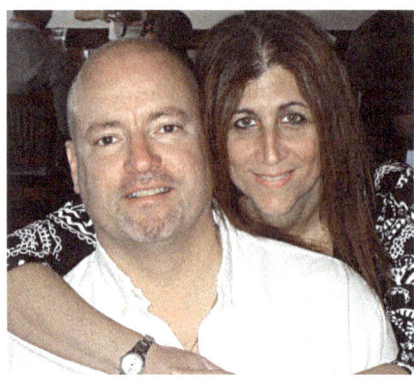

Heidi and Bill, Ruth's niece and nephew.

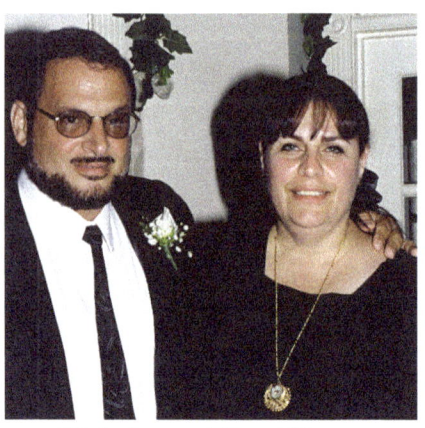

Nicholas and Terri Vuoto.

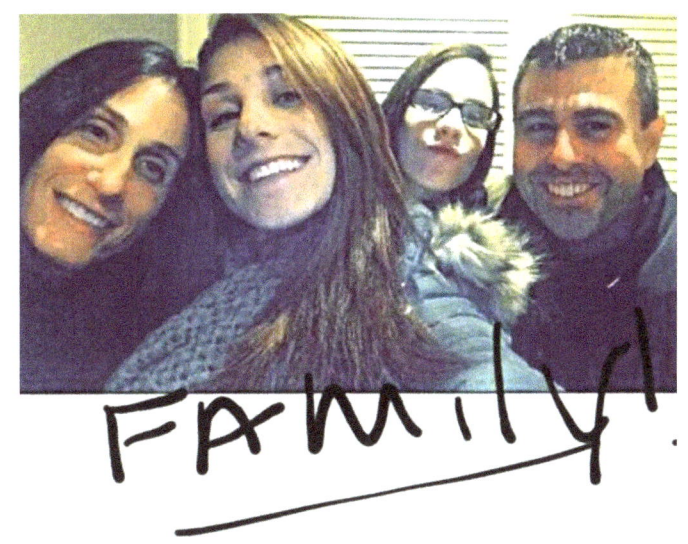

Jamie, Dani, Kati Rose, and Rob,
Ruth's grandchildren.

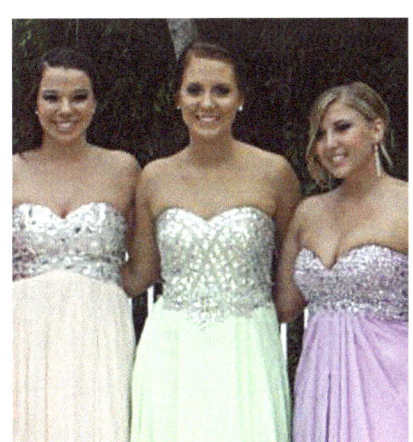

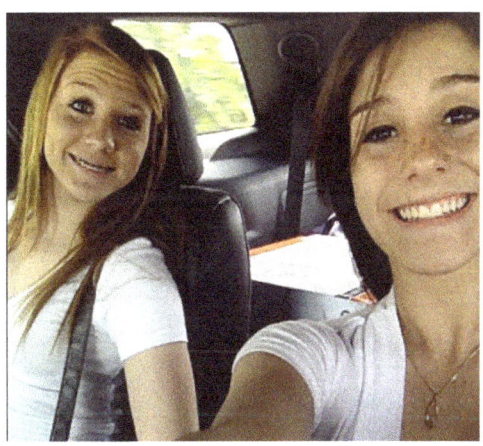

Casey, center.   *Casey and Dani Nic.*

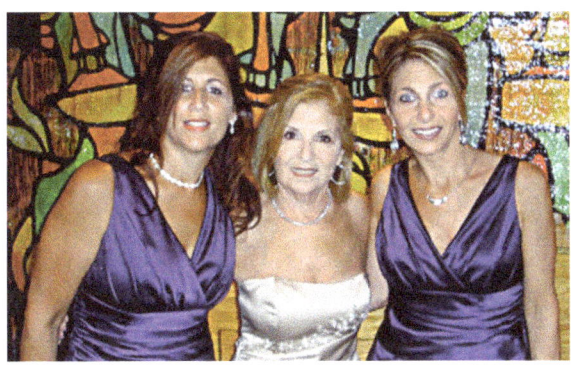

Heidi, Carol and Annie, Ruth's nieces.

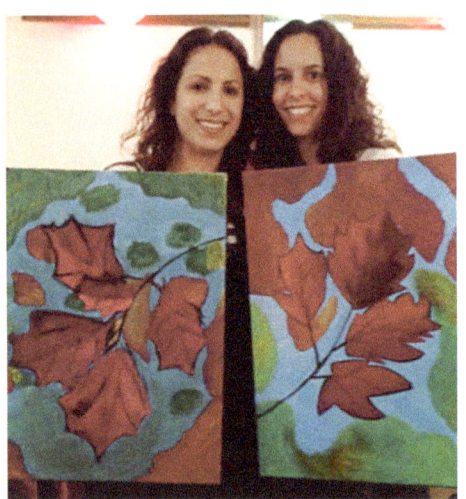

Andrea and Nicole.

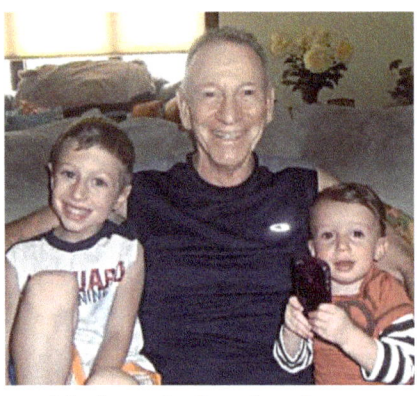

Nephew Arthur Landman.

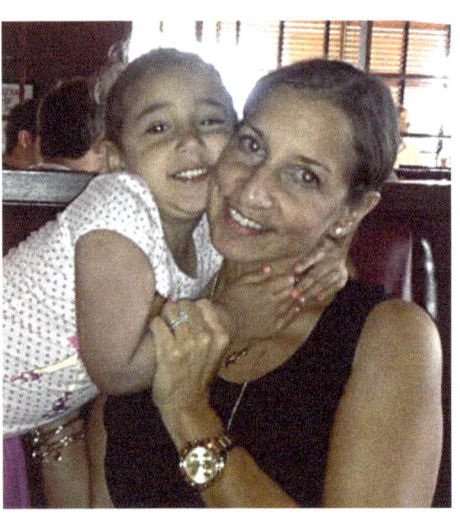

Nieces Karyn and Emersyn.

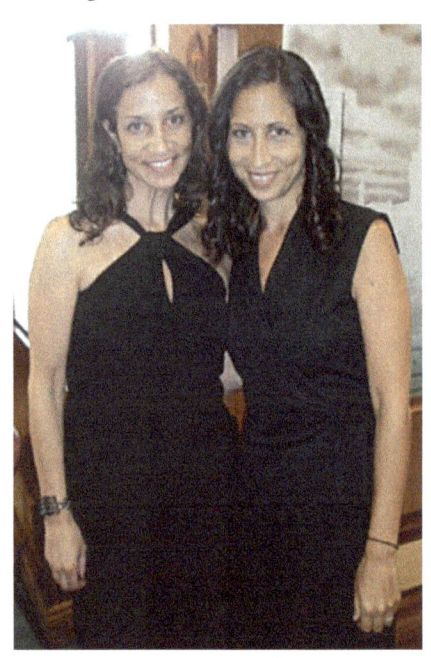

Nieces Karyn and Dayna.

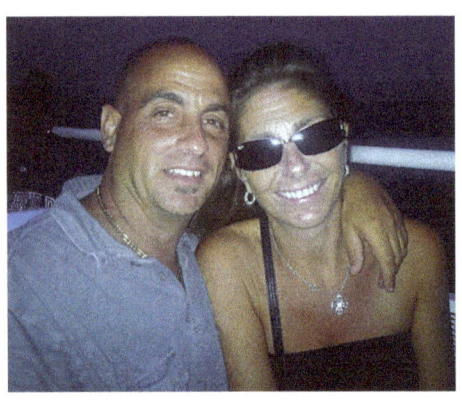

Michael and Annie.

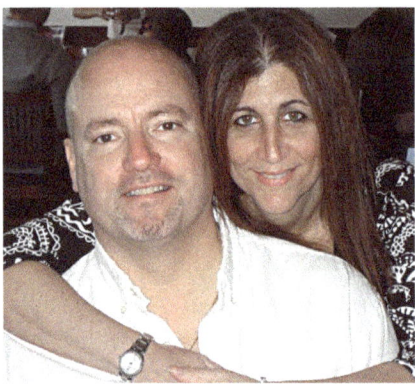

Heidi and Bill, niece and nephew.

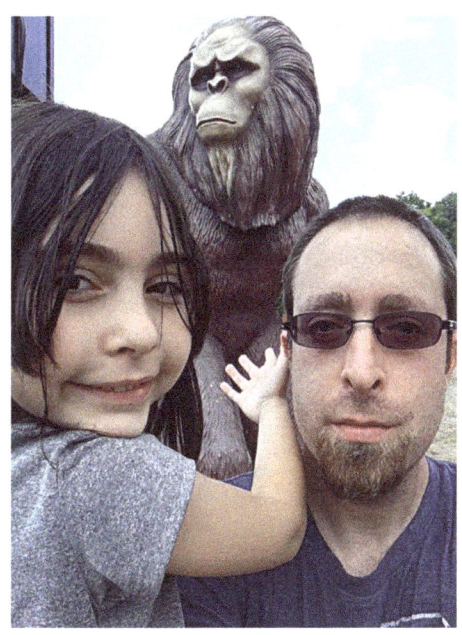

Penelope and Jared.

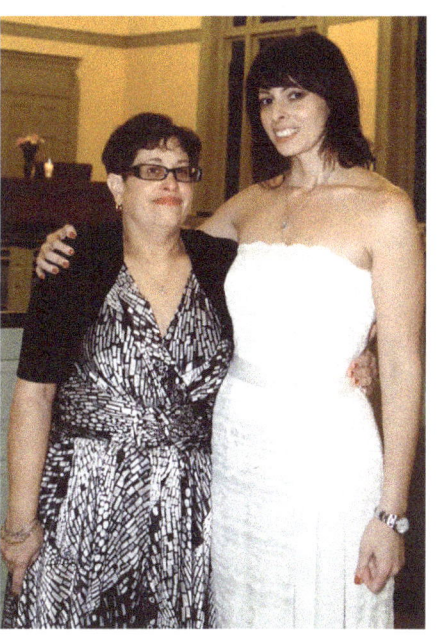

Susan and Faith, Ruth's nieces.

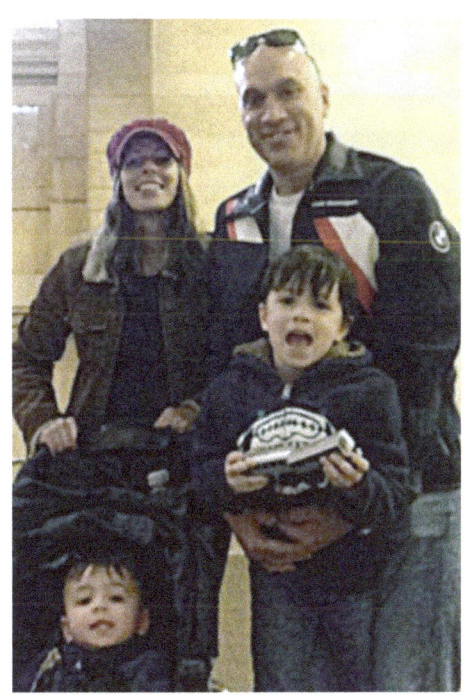

Faith, Chris, CW and RT, Ruth's niece and nephews

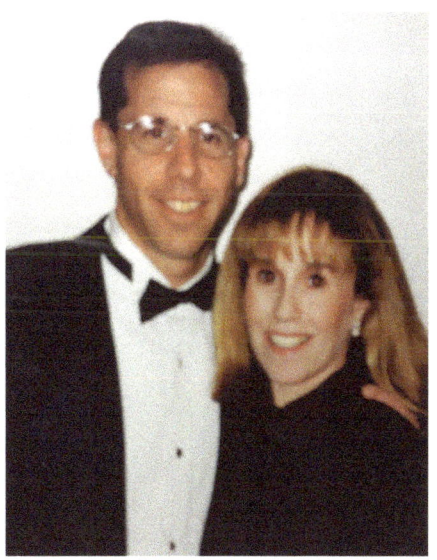

Ruth's son, Keith, and his wife, Marcia.

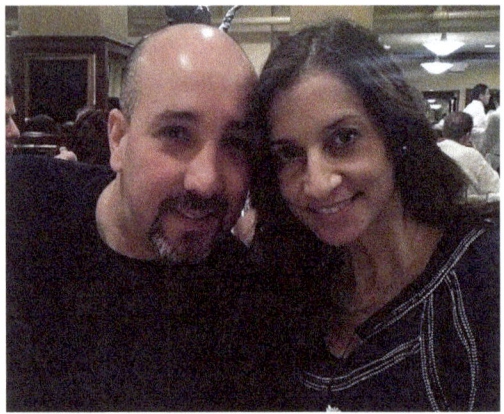

Karyn and Randy, Ruth's nephew and niece.

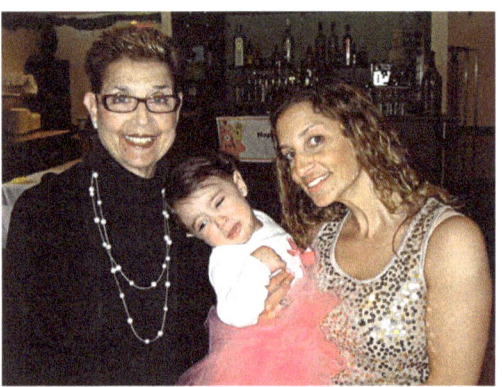

Fran Landman andKaryn, Ruth's nieces, wtih Emersyn.

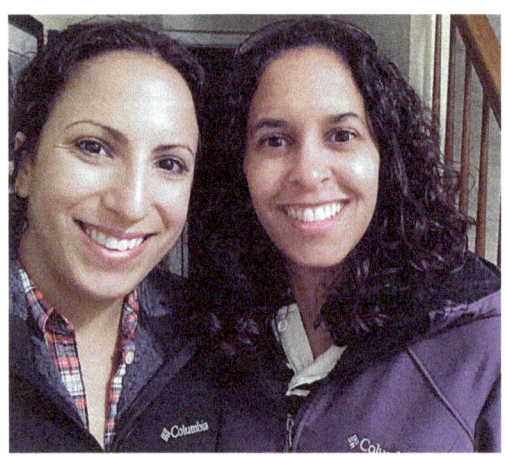

Andrea and Nicole.

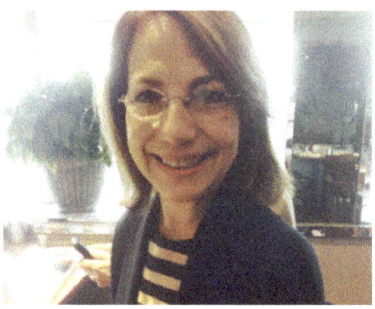

Phyllis, Ruth's niece.

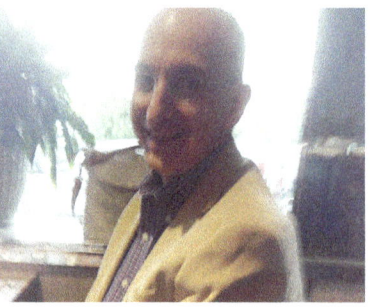

Ken.

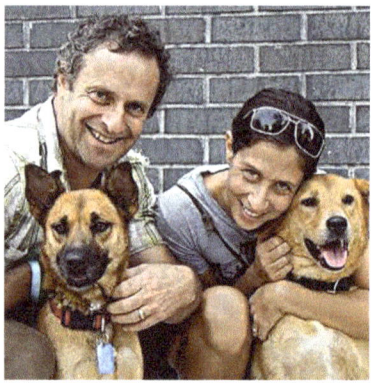

Dayna and Michel, Ruth's niece and nephew.

I Dare You to Stop Me… The Challenge is On!

I am the voice of Alzheimer's and let me tell you this … my boundaries are limitless. I can strike anyone at anytime. I am not partial to race, creed or gender. I travel all over the world. I live in the minds of people in every village, town, city, state, country, and continent in the entire world. If I could invade outer space, I would.

My goal, unless you stop me, is to take over and rule as many minds as possible, increasing the need for more nursing homes and home health aides, while draining Medicare and Medicaid services. I hope to use up all of your resources … unless you stop me and FIND A CURE!

I challenge you—all of you researchers and doctors—to find a cure and stop me from spreading.

CPSIA information can be obtained
at www.ICGtesting.com
Printed in the USA
LVHW07s1516160818
587180LV00037B/1087/P